Drugs of Choice

Selected Articles from *Treatment Guidelines*
with updates from *The Medical Letter*®

Published by

The Medical Letter, Inc.
145 Huguenot St.
New Rochelle, New York 10801-7537

800-211-2769
914-235-0500
Fax 914-632-1733
www.medicalletter.org

18th Edition

Copyright 2012
(ISSN 1065-6596)
(ISBN 978-0-9815278-6-4)

The Medical Letter Inc.
145 Huguenot St., Ste. 312
New Rochelle, New York 10801-7537

Contents

Tables

EDITOR IN CHIEF: Mark Abramowicz, M.D.
EXECUTIVE EDITOR: Gianna Zuccotti, M.D., M.P.H., F.A.C.P., Harvard
Medical School
EDITOR: Jean-Marie Pflomm, Pharm.D.

ASSISTANT EDITORS, DRUG INFORMATION: Susan M. Daron, Pharm.D.,
Corinne E. Zanone, Pharm.D.

CONSULTING EDITORS: Brinda M. Shah, Pharm.D., **F. Peter Swanson**, M.D.

CONTRIBUTING EDITORS:
Carl W. Bazil, M.D., Ph.D., Columbia University College of Physicians and
Surgeons
Vanessa K. Dalton, M.D., M.P.H., University of Michigan Medical School
Eric J. Epstein, M.D., Albert Einstein College of Medicine
Jules Hirsch, M.D., Rockefeller University
David N. Juurlink, BPhm, M.D., Ph.D., Sunnybrook Health Sciences Centre
Richard B. Kim, M.D., University of Western Ontario
Hans Meinertz, M.D., University Hospital, Copenhagen
Sandip K. Mukherjee, M.D., F.A.C.C., Yale School of Medicine
Dan M. Roden, M.D., Vanderbilt University School of Medicine
F. Estelle R. Simons, M.D., University of Manitoba
Jordan W. Smoller, M.D., Sc.D., Harvard Medical School
Neal H. Steigbigel, M.D., New York University School of Medicine
Arthur M. F. Yee, M.D., Ph.D., F.A.C.R., Weil Medical College of Cornell
University

SENIOR ASSOCIATE EDITORS: Donna Goodstein, Amy Faucard
ASSOCIATE EDITOR: Cynthia Macapagal Covey

EDITORIAL FELLOW: Esperance A.K. Schaefer, M.D., M.P.H., Harvard
Medical School

MANAGING EDITOR: Susie Wong
ASSISTANT MANAGING EDITOR: Liz Donohue
PRODUCTION COORDINATOR: Cheryl Brown

EXECUTIVE DIRECTOR OF SALES: Gene Carbona
FULFILLMENT & SYSTEMS MANAGER: Cristine Romatowski
DIRECTOR OF MARKETING COMMUNICATIONS: Joanne F. Valentino
VICE PRESIDENT AND PUBLISHER: Yosef Wissner-Levy

Introduction

The Medical Letter, Inc. is a nonprofit company founded in 1958 by Arthur Kallet, the co-founder of Consumers Union, and Dr. Harold Aaron, with the goal of providing healthcare professionals with objective, independent analyses of both prescription and over-the-counter drugs. In addition to its newsletters, *The Medical Letter on Drugs and Therapeutics* and *Treatment Guidelines from The Medical Letter*, the company also publishes handbooks and software on topics such as antimicrobial therapy and drug interactions. It is supported solely by subscription fees and accepts no advertising, grants or donations.

The Medical Letter on Drugs and Therapeutics offers comprehensive drug evaluations of virtually all new drugs and reviews of older drugs when important new information becomes available on their usefulness or adverse effects. Occasionally, *The Medical Letter* publishes an article on a new non-drug treatment or a diagnostic aid. *Treatment Guidelines from The Medical Letter* consists of review articles of drug classes for treatment of major indications. A typical issue contains recommendations for first choice and alternative drugs with assessments of the drugs' effectiveness and safety. *The Medical Letter* is published every other week and *Treatment Guidelines* is published once a month. Both are intended to meet the needs of the busy healthcare professional who wants unbiased, reliable and timely information on new drugs and comprehensive reviews of treatments of choice for major indications. Both publications help healthcare professionals make decisions based on the best interests of their patients, rather than the commercial interests of the pharmaceutical industry.

The editorial process used for Medical Letter publications relies on a consensus of experts to develop prescribing recommendations. An expert reviewer, one of our editors, or one of our contributing editors prepares the preliminary report on a drug (for *The Medical Letter*) or drugs for common disorders (for *Treatment Guidelines*) in terms of their effectiveness, adverse effects and possible alternatives. Both published and available unpublished studies are carefully examined, paying special attention to the results of controlled clinical trials. The preliminary draft is edited and sent to our contributing editors, to 10-20 other investigators who have clinical and experimental experience with the drug or type of drug or disease under review, to the FDA and, if applicable, to the CDC, and to the first authors of all the articles cited in the text.

Many critical observations, suggestions and questions are received from the reviewers and are incorporated into the article during the revision process. Further communication as needed is followed by checking and editing to make sure the final appraisal is not only accurate, but also easy to read.

The Medical Letter, Inc., is based in New Rochelle, NY. For more information go to www.medicalletter.org or call (800) 211-2769.

DRUGS FOR
Allergic Disorders

Original publication date – February 2010 (revised March 2012)

Allergic rhinitis, allergic conjunctivitis, atopic dermatitis, urticaria, ana-phylaxis and asthma (not included here; reviewed in *Treatment Guide-lines* 2012; 10:11. See page 51) are prevalent worldwide, especially in industrialized countries. Pharmacologic treatment of these disorders con-tinues to improve in efficacy and safety. In addition to using drugs to pre-vent and control these allergic diseases, patients should be instructed to avoid, if possible, specific allergens and/or environmental conditions that trigger or worsen their symptoms. Allergen-specific immunotherapy may be useful for treatment of allergic rhinitis and allergic conjunctivitis, and in preventing severe insect venom-triggered reactions.

ALLERGIC RHINITIS

Allergic rhinitis may be seasonal/intermittent or perennial/persistent. H_1-antihistamines, the drugs most commonly used to treat this disorder, are more effective in relieving sneezing, itching and discharge than in reliev-ing nasal congestion.[1]

H_1-Antihistamines – First-generation H_1-antihistamines such as diphenhydramine (*Benadryl*, and others) or chlorpheniramine (*Chlor-Trimeton*, and others) are inexpensive, but even in usual doses they may cause somnolence, interfere with learning and memory, decrease work

1

SOME ORAL DRUGS FOR ALLERGIC RHINITIS

Drug	Formulations
ORAL SECOND-GENERATION H$_1$-ANTIHISTAMINES	
Cetirizine[1] – generic *Zyrtec* (McNeil Consumer)	5, 10 mg chew tabs; 10 mg tabs; 1 mg/1 mL syrup
Cetirizine/pseudoephedrine[1] generic *Zyrtec-D 12 hour* (McNeil Consumer)	5 mg/120 mg ER tabs
Desloratadine – *Clarinex* (Schering-Plough)	5 mg tabs; 0.5 mg/mL syrup 2.5, 5 mg disintegrating tabs
Desloratadine/pseudoephedrine *Clarinex-D 12 hour* (Schering-Plough) *Clarinex-D 24 hour*	2.5 mg/120 mg ER tabs 5 mg/240 mg ER tabs
Fexofenadine[1] – generic *Allegra* (Sanofi-aventis, PD-RX)	30, 60, 180 mg tabs 60, 180 mg tab; 30 mg/5 mL susp; 30 mg disintegrating tab
Fexofenadine/pseudoephedrine[1] *Allegra-D 12 hour* (Sanofi-aventis, and others) *Allegra-D 24 hour*	60 mg/120 mg ER tabs 180 mg/240 mg ER tabs
Levocetirizine – *Xyzal* (Sanofi-aventis, UCB)	5 mg tabs; 0.5 mg/mL oral solution
Loratadine[1] – generic *Claritin* (Schering-Plough) *Alavert* (Wyeth)	10 mg tabs; 10 mg disintegrating tabs; 1 mg/mL syrup and susp 10 mg tabs; 1 mg/mL syrup; 5, 10 mg disintegrating tabs;10 mg caps 10 mg tabs; 10 mg disintegrating tabs

1. Available without a prescription.
2. Only approved for treatment of chronic idiopathic urticaria and perennial allergic rhinitis in this age group.

Usual Daily Adult Dosage	Usual Daily Pediatric Dosage
5 or 10 mg 1x/d	6-11 mos: 2.5 mg 1x/d[2] 12-23 mos: 2.5 mg 1x/d-bid[2] 2-5 yrs: 2.5 or 5 mg 1x/d or 2.5 mg bid 6-11 yrs: 5-10 mg 1x/d
1 tab bid	≥12 yrs: 1 tab bid
5 mg 1x/d	6-23 mos: 1 mg 1x/d[3] 2-5 yrs: 1.25 mg 1x/d 6-11 yrs: 2.5 mg 1x/d
1 tab bid	≥12 yrs: 1 tab bid
1 tab 1x/d	≥12 yrs: 1 tab 1x/d
60 mg bid or 180 mg 1x/d	6-23 mos: 15 mg bid[3] 2-11 yrs: 30 mg bid
1 tab bid	≥12 yrs: 1 tab bid
1 tab 1x/d	≥12 yrs: 1 tab 1x/d
5 mg 1x/d	6 mos-5 yrs: 1.25 mg 1x/d[4] 6-11 yrs: 2.5 mg 1x/d
10 mg 1x/d	2-5 yrs: 5 mg 1x/d ≥6 yrs: 10 mg 1x/d

3. Only approved for treatment of chronic idiopathic urticaria in this age group.
4. Not approved for treatment of seasonal allergic rhinitis in children <2 years old.

Continued on next page.

SOME ORAL DRUGS FOR ALLERGIC RHINITIS (continued)

Drug	Formulations
ORAL SECOND-GENERATION H$_1$-ANTIHISTAMINES (continued)	
Loratadine/pseudoephedrine[1]	
Claritin-D 12 hour (Schering-Plough)	5 mg/120 mg ER tabs
Claritin-D 24 hour	10 mg/240 mg ER tabs
Alavert-D 12 hour (Wyeth)	5 mg/120 mg ER tabs
LEUKOTRIENE RECEPTOR ANTAGONIST	
Montelukast – *Singulair* (Merck)	10 mg tabs; 4, 5 mg chew tabs; 4 mg granule packets

productivity, impair performance on examinations and other cognitive activities, and increase the risk of on-the-job injuries.[2]

First-generation antihistamines cause CNS adverse effects because they penetrate the blood-brain barrier, bind to H$_1$-receptors in the brain and interfere with the neurotransmitter effects of histamine. The patient may be unaware of these effects, which can persist in the morning after taking the drug at bedtime and may continue to occur with regular use. First-generation H$_1$-antihistamines also cause anticholinergic effects such as dry mouth and urinary retention. Administration of the first-generation H$_1$-antihistamine promethazine (*Phenergan*, and others) to infants and children <2 years old has been associated with respiratory depression and death. Mixtures containing first-generation H$_1$-antihistamines sold for the relief of cough, colds, allergies and insomnia are no longer approved in the US for children <2 years old or in Canada for children <6 years old. There are also concerns about use of first-generation H$_1$-antihistamines in the elderly because of their potential for adverse effects and drug-drug interactions.[3]

Usual Daily Adult Dosage	Usual Daily Pediatric Dosage
1 tab bid	≥12 yrs: 1 tab bid
1 tab 1x/d	≥12 yrs: 1 tab 1x/d
1 tab bid	≥12 yrs: 1 tab bid
10 mg 1x/d	6 mos-5 yrs: 4 mg 1x/d
	6-14 yrs: 5 mg 1x/d

Second-generation H_1-antihistamines are used as first-line therapy in patients with mild to moderate allergic rhinitis. They penetrate poorly into the brain and are significantly less likely to have CNS adverse effects than first-generation antihistamines. Fexofenadine is free of sedative effects, even in higher-than-recommended doses. Loratadine and desloratadine (an active metabolite of loratadine) are nonsedating in recommended doses; sedation may occur with higher doses. Cetirizine is potentially more sedating than some other second-generation agents. The long-term safety of cetirizine, levocetirizine and loratadine in young children is better established than that of other first- or second-generation antihistamines. It is not clear that levocetirizine offers any advantage over cetirizine.[4,5]

Topical intranasal H_1-antihistamines have a rapid onset of action and are well tolerated. Their clinical efficacy in allergic rhinitis, including some beneficial effects on nasal congestion, appears to be equal or superior to that of oral second-generation H_1-antihistamines.[6,7]

SOME NASAL SPRAYS FOR ALLERGIC RHINITIS

Drug	Formulations
H_1-ANTIHISTAMINE	
Azelastine – *Astelin* 0.1%(Meda)	Metered-dose pump spray (137 mcg/spray)
Astepro 0.1% (Meda)[1]	Metered-dose pump spray (137 mcg/spray)
Astepro 0.15%	Metered-dose pump spray (205.5 mcg/spray)
Olopatadine – *Patanase* (Alcon)	Metered-dose pump spray (665 mcg/spray)
CORTICOSTEROIDS	
Beclomethasone dipropionate *Beconase AQ* (GSK)	Metered-dose pump spray (42 mcg/spray)
Budesonide – *Rhinocort Aqua* (Astra Zeneca)	Metered-dose pump spray (32 mcg/spray)
Ciclesonide – *Omnaris* (Sepracor/Nycomed)	Metered-dose pump spray (50 mcg/spray)
Flunisolide generic	Metered-dose pump spray (25 mcg/spray)
Fluticasone furoate – *Veramyst* (GSK)	Metered-dose pump spray (27.5 mcg/spray)
Fluticasone propionate generic *Flonase* (GSK)	Metered-dose pump spray (50 mcg/spray)
Mometasone furoate *Nasonex* (Schering-Plough)	Metered-dose pump spray (50 mcg/spray)
Triamcinolone acetonide *Nasacort AQ* (Sanofi-Aventis)	Metered-dose pump spray (55 mcg/spray)

1. FDA approved for the treatment of seasonal allergic rhinitis.
2. Dosage for seasonal allergic rhinitis is 1-2 sprays per nostril bid or 2 sprays per nostril once daily.
   Dosage for perennial allergic rhinitis is 2 sprays per nostril bid.

Usual Daily Adult Dosage	Usual Daily Pediatric Dosage
1-2 sprays per nostril 2x/d	5-11 yrs: 1 spray per nostril 2x/d
1-2 sprays per nostril 2x/d	$\geq$12 yrs: 1-2 sprays per nostril 2x/d
1-2 sprays per nostril 2x/d[2]	$\geq$12 yrs: 1-2 sprays per nostril 1-2x/d
2 sprays per nostril 2x/d	$\geq$12 yrs: 2 sprays per nostril 2x/d
1-2 sprays per nostril 2x/d	$\geq$6 yrs: 1-2 sprays per nostril 2x/d
1-4 sprays per nostril 1x/d	6-11 yrs: 1-2 sprays per nostril 1x/d
2 sprays per nostril 1x/d	$\geq$6 yrs[3]: 2 sprays per nostril 1x/d
2 sprays per nostril bid-tid	6-14 yrs: 1 spray per nostril tid or 2 sprays per nostril 2x/d
2 sprays per nostril 1x/d	2-11 yrs: 1-2 sprays per nostril 1x/d
1-2 sprays per nostril 1x/d or 1 spray per nostril 2x/d	$\geq$4 yrs: 1-2 sprays per nostril 1x/d
2 sprays per nostril 1x/d	2-11 yrs: 1-2 sprays per nostril 1x/d
2 sprays per nostril 1x/d	2-5 yrs: 1 spray per nostril 1x/d 6-11 yrs: 1-2 sprays per nostril 1x/d

3. Not approved for treatment of perennial allergic rhinitis in children <12 years old.

Continued on next page.

SOME NASAL SPRAYS FOR ALLERGIC RHINITIS (continued)

Drug	Formulations
MAST-CELL STABILIZER	
Cromolyn sodium – *Nasalcrom*[4] (Pfizer Consumer)	Metered-dose pump spray (5.2 mg/spray)
ANTICHOLINERGIC	
Ipratropium bromide	Metered-dose pump spray
generic	(21 or 42 mcg/spray)
Atrovent (Boehringer Ingelheim)	(21 or 42 mcg/spray)

4. Available without a prescription.

Intranasal Corticosteroids – Topical intranasal corticosteroids are the most effective drugs available for prevention and relief of allergic rhinitis symptoms and are the drugs of choice for treatment of moderate to severe disease. All of these agents reduce sneezing, itching, discharge and congestion. Most are effective when given once daily. There is no clear dose-response relationship with these drugs, suggesting that currently recommended doses are already at the plateau of the dose-response curve. Although the onset of action generally occurs within 12 hours, they may take 7 days or more to be maximally effective. Intranasal corticosteroid sprays may be effective in decreasing ocular as well as nasal symptoms of seasonal allergic rhinitis.[8,9]

Adverse effects of intranasal corticosteroid treatment are mild; they include dryness and irritation, burning or bleeding of the nasal mucosa, sore throat, epistaxis and headache. Sensory attributes of intranasal corticosteroid formulations such as odor and aftertaste may affect patient compliance.[10]

Intranasal corticosteroids used as directed generally do not cause atrophy of the nasal mucosa. Growth suppression has been reported with use of intranasal beclomethasone dipropionate bid for 12 months in children 6-9

Usual Daily Adult Dosage	Usual Daily Pediatric Dosage
1 spray per nostril tid-qid	≥2 yrs: 1 spray per nostril tid-qid
2 sprays per nostril bid-qid	≥5 yrs: 2 sprays per nostril bid-qid

years old, but not with newer intranasal corticosteroids such as ciclesonide, fluticasone propionate or mometasone.[11] Because many patients may require long-term treatment with corticosteroids by various routes (intranasal for rhinitis, inhaled orally for asthma, and applied topically for atopic dermatitis), it is important with all routes to prescribe the lowest dose that prevents and controls symptoms.

Leukotriene Receptor Antagonist – Cysteinyl leukotrienes are released in the nasal mucosa during allergic inflammation and produce nasal congestion. Montelukast *(Singulair)*, the only leukotriene receptor antagonist FDA-approved for use in seasonal and perennial allergic rhinitis, has a modest effect in relieving sneezing, itching, discharge and congestion, but it is less effective than intranasal corticosteroids. The combination of a leukotriene receptor antagonist and an H_1-antihistamine is superior to either used alone.

Decongestants – Decongestants act as vasoconstrictors in the nasal mucosa primarily through stimulation of alpha-1 adrenergic receptors on venous sinusoids. They are effective only for relief of congestion, and not for sneezing, itching or discharge. Some oral formulations containing pseudoephedrine are being removed from the market because of concerns about illicit use. Substitutes containing phenylephrine (*Sudafed PE*, and others) may not be effective.[12]

Adverse effects of oral decongestants include insomnia, excitability, headache, nervousness, anorexia, palpitations, tachycardia, arrhythmias, hypertension, nausea, vomiting and urinary retention. Pseudoephedrine should be used cautiously in patients with cardiovascular disease, hypertension, diabetes, hyperthyroidism, closed-angle glaucoma or bladder neck obstruction.

Topical intranasal decongestants are less likely than oral drugs to cause systemic effects, but they may cause stinging, burning, sneezing and dryness of the nose and throat. In order to avoid rebound congestion, they should not be used for more than three consecutive days. Rhinitis medicamentosa associated with prolonged use of topical drugs is treated by discontinuing the topical decongestant and administering intranasal corticosteroids to control symptoms.[13]

Mast-Cell Stabilizer – Cromolyn sodium, given before allergen exposure, inhibits mast cell degranulation and mediator release. It is sometimes used for prophylaxis of allergic rhinitis symptoms, but is considerably less effective than intranasal corticosteroids and must be used 4 times a day. Cromolyn sodium has virtually no local or systemic toxicity.

Anticholinergic – Ipratropium bromide is a quaternary amine antimuscarinic agent. Given as a nasal spray, it is poorly absorbed systemically and does not readily cross the blood-brain barrier. Ipratropium is useful in patients whose primary symptom is nasal discharge, for example after exposure to irritants or cold air, or as an adjunct to reduce rhinorrhea not controlled by other medications. It does not relieve sneezing, itching or nasal congestion. Ipratropium may cause dry nose and mouth, pharyngeal irritation, urinary retention and, with inadvertent instillation in the eye, increases in intraocular pressure. It should be used with caution in patients with glaucoma and in those with prostatic hypertrophy or bladder neck obstruction.

Omalizumab (Anti-IgE Antibody) – Omalizumab *(Xolair)*, which is injected subcutaneously for treatment of allergic asthma,[14] decreases free IgE levels in serum, the number of IgE receptors on mast cells and basophils, and the nasal response to allergens. It has a dose-dependent beneficial effect in seasonal allergic rhinitis; how its efficacy compares to that of H_1-antihistamines and intranasal corticosteroids remains to be determined. Omalizumab is generally well tolerated, but rarely causes anaphylaxis. It has not been approved by the FDA for treatment of allergic rhinitis.

Systemic Corticosteroids – Patients with severe allergic rhinitis who do not respond to, or are intolerant of, other drugs are sometimes treated with oral corticosteroids, a last resort that should be avoided if possible.

Complementary and Alternative Treatments – Herbal remedies, homeopathy and acupuncture are widely used for allergic rhinitis symptoms, but their efficacy has not been established.[15]

Pregnancy – Drugs used in allergic rhinitis for which safety in pregnancy has been demonstrated include intranasal corticosteroids, the H_1-antihistamines cetirizine and loratadine, the topical ophthalmic H_1-antihistamine emedastine, the leukotriene receptor antagonist montelukast and the mast-cell stabilizer cromolyn sodium.

Drugs of Choice – For mild to moderate allergic rhinitis, especially for seasonal or intermittent symptoms, an oral second-generation H_1-antihistamine or an intranasal H_1-antihistamine is a reasonable choice. For moderate to severe allergic rhinitis, an intranasal corticosteroid is more likely to be effective. No single oral second-generation H_1-antihistamine or intranasal corticosteroid has been convincingly demonstrated to be superior to any other within the same class.

Drugs for Allergic Disorders

SOME OPHTHALMIC DRUGS FOR ALLERGIC CONJUNCTIVITIS

Drug	Some Formulations
H_1-ANTIHISTAMINES	
Emedastine difumarate	0.05% soln*
Emadine (Alcon)	
MAST-CELL STABILIZERS	
Cromolyn sodium[1] – generic	4% soln*
Lodoxamide tromethamine	
Alomide[1] (Alcon)	0.1% soln*
Nedocromil	
Alocril (Allergan)	2% soln*
Pemirolast potassium	
Alamast (Vistakon)	0.1% soln**
H_1-ANTIHISTAMINES AND MAST-CELL STABILIZERS	
Alcaftadine	
Lastacaft (Allergan)	0.25% soln*
Azelastine	
Optivar (Meda)	0.05% soln*
Bepotastine	
Bepreve (Ista)	1.5% soln*
Epinastine	
Elestat (Allergan)	0.05% soln*
Ketotifen fumarate[2] – generic	0.025% soln*
Zaditor (Novartis)	0.025% soln*
Claritin Eye (Schering-Plough)	0.025% soln*
Eye Itch Relief (Major)	0.025% soln*
Olopatadine – *Pataday* (Alcon)	0.2% soln*
Patanol (Alcon)	0.1% soln*
NONSTEROIDAL ANTI-INFLAMMATORY DRUGS (NSAIDs)	
Ketorolac tromethamine – generic	0.5% soln*[3]
Acular (Allergan)	

* Contains benzalkonium chloride. ** Contains lauralkonium chloride, which may cause irritation.
1. Approved by the FDA for treatment of vernal keratoconjunctivitis, vernal conjunctivitis and vernal keratitis.

12

Available Sizes	Usual Daily Dosage	Pediatric Age Range
5 mL	1 drop qid	$\geq$3 yrs
10 mL	1-2 drops q4-6h	>4 yrs
10 mL	1 drop qid	>2 yrs
5 mL	1-2 drops bid	>3 yrs
10 mL	1-2 drops qid	$\geq$3 yrs
3 mL	1 drop 1x/d	>2 yrs
6 mL	1 drop bid	$\geq$3 yrs
10 mL	1 drop bid	$\geq$2 yrs
5 mL	1 drop bid	$\geq$3 yrs
5 mL	1 drop q8-12h	$\geq$3 yrs
5 mL	1 drop q8-12h	$\geq$3 yrs
5 mL	1 drop q8-12h	$\geq$3 yrs
5 mL	1 drop q8-12h	$\geq$3 yrs
2.5 mL	1 drop 1x/d	$\geq$3 yrs
5 mL	1-2 drops bid	$\geq$3 yrs
3, 5, 10 mL	1 drop qid	$\geq$3 yrs

2. Available over the counter.
3. Also available in 0.4% soln for use in incisional refractive surgery.

ALLERGIC CONJUNCTIVITIS

Allergic conjunctivitis, the most common form of ocular allergy, is often associated with seasonal allergic rhinitis. The main symptom, itching, is usually relieved by an **oral H_1-antihistamine**, preferably a second-generation, minimally or nonsedating drug such as cetirizine, desloratadine, fexofenadine, levocetirizine or loratadine.[16] **Antihistamine eye drops** are also effective, and have a more rapid onset of action (within a few minutes). Ketotifen (which is available over the counter), azelastine, bepotastine, epinastine and olopatadine are marketed as having both H_1-antihistamine and mast-cell-stabilizing activity, but all H_1-antihistamines probably have some mast-cell-stabilizing activity. Ophthalmic **stabilizers** cromolyn, lodoxamide, nedocromil and pemirolast have a slower onset of action than H_1-antihistamines, and are mostly used for treatment of mild to moderate symptoms.[17] The topical nonsteroidal anti-inflammatory drug ketorolac can also be used, but in comparative studies it was less effective than olopatadine or emedastine.[18]

Topical ophthalmic decongestants reduce erythema, congestion, itching and eyelid edema, but are not drugs of choice because of their short duration of action and adverse effects, including burning, stinging, rebound hyperemia and conjunctivitis medicamentosa. Because of these effects, **antihistamine/decongestant combination eye drops** available over the counter such as pheniramine/naphazoline (*Visine A*, and others) and antazoline/naphazoline (*Vasocon-A*) are not good choices either, except for very short-term use in mild disease.

Patients who find that application of any topical ophthalmic preparation leads to stinging or burning should try refrigerating the drug before use. **Intranasal corticosteroid sprays** may also help relieve symptoms of allergic conjunctivitis.[19]

Topical **ophthalmic corticosteroids** should be considered a last resort in extreme situations. A corticosteroid that is inactivated rapidly in the anterior chamber, such as rimexolone (*Vexol*) or low-dose loteprednol etabonate (*Alrex, Lotemax*), is preferred. Duration of treatment should be limited to 1-2 weeks. The patient should be monitored by an ophthalmologist because these medications have been associated with exacerbations of viral infections of the conjunctiva and cornea, increased intraocular pressure and cataract formation.

Drugs of Choice – Any second-generation oral H_1-antihistamine or topical ophthalmic H_1-antihistamine/mast-cell stabilizer is effective and safe for the treatment of allergic conjunctivitis.

ATOPIC DERMATITIS

Treatment of atopic dermatitis/eczema includes hydration and moisturization, topical anti-inflammatory agents such as corticosteroids and calcineurin inhibitors, as well as anti-infective therapy.[20]

Topical Corticosteroids – A medium- or high-potency topical corticosteroid may be needed to control skin inflammation in atopic dermatitis, but for maintenance treatment the topical corticosteroid with the lowest potency that is effective in a given patient should be used. High-potency corticosteroids such as betamethasone dipropionate 0.05% ointment/cream should never be used on the face; even on the trunk and extremities, they should be used only for short periods of time. Low-potency corticosteroids such as hydrocortisone cream can be used safely on the face and intertriginous areas.

Local adverse effects of topical corticosteroids include development of striae and skin atrophy. Used on the eyelids for prolonged periods, they can cause glaucoma and cataracts. Systemic side effects relate to corticosteroid potency, site of application, percentage of body surface covered and duration of treatment. The potential for adrenal suppression is greatest with high-potency corticosteroids or when corticosteroids are applied under occlusive dressings, especially in infants and young children with

Continued on page 20

SOME TOPICAL DRUGS FOR ATOPIC DERMATITIS

Drug	Vehicle
CALCINEURIN INHIBITORS	
Pimecrolimus 1%	
Elidel (Novartis)	cream
Tacrolimus 0.03%	
Protopic (Astellas)	oint
Tacrolimus 0.1%	
Protopic (Astellas)	oint
CORTICOSTEROIDS	
Super-High Potency	
Betamethasone dipropionate	
augmented 0.05% – generic	oint, lotion, gel
Diprolene (Schering-Plough)	oint, gel
Clobetasol propionate 0.05%	
generic	cream, oint, gel, foam, soln
Cormax (Watson)	oint, soln
Clobex (Galderma)	lotion, spray, shampoo
Olux (Connetics Corp)	foam
Temovate (GSK)	cream, soln, oint, gel
Fluocinonide 0.1%	
Vanos (Medicis)	cream
Halobetasol propionate 0.05%	
generic	cream, oint
Ultravate (Ranbaxy)	cream, oint
High Potency	
Amcinonide 0.1% – generic	oint
Betamethasone dipropionate 0.05%	
augmented – generic	cream
Diprolene AF (Schering-Plough)	cream
Betamethasone dipropionate 0.05%	
generic	oint

SOME TOPICAL DRUGS FOR ATOPIC DERMATITIS (continued)

Drug	Vehicle
High Potency (continued)	
Desoximetasone 0.25%	
generic	cream, gel, oint
Topicort (Taro)	cream, gel, oint
Desoximetasone 0.05%	
generic	gel
Topicort 0.05% (Taro)	gel
Diflorasone diacetate 0.05%	
generic	oint
Fluocinonide 0.05%	
generic	gel, oint, soln, cream
Halcinonide 0.1%	
Halog (Ranbaxy)	cream, oint
Mometasone furoate 0.1%	
generic	oint
Elocon (Schering-Plough)	oint
Triamcinolone acetonide 0.5%	
generic	oint
Medium-High Potency	
Amcinonide 0.1%	
generic	cream, lotion
Betamethasone dipropionate 0.05%	
generic	cream
Betamethasone	
valerate 0.1% – generic	oint
Desoximetasone 0.05%	
generic	cream
Diflorasone	
diacetate 0.05%	
generic	cream
Fluocinonide	
emollient 0.05%	
generic	cream

Continued on next page.

SOME TOPICAL DRUGS FOR ATOPIC DERMATITIS (continued)

Drug	Vehicle
Medium-High Potency (continued)	
Fluticasone propionate 0.005%	
generic	oint
Cutivate (PharmDerm)	
Triamcinolone	
acetonide 0.1%	
generic	oint
Triamcinolone acetonide 0.5%	
generic	cream
Medium Potency	
Betamethasone valerate 0.12%	
Luxiq (Stiefel Labs)	foam
Fluocinolone	
acetonide 0.025%	
generic	oint
Hydrocortisone	
valerate 0.2%	
generic	oint
Westcort (Ranbaxy)	oint
Mometasone furoate 0.1%	
generic	cream, lotion
Elocon (Schering-Plough)	cream, lotion
Triamcinolone acetonide 0.1%	
generic	cream
Medium-Low Potency	
Betamethasone dipropionate 0.05%	
generic	lotion
Betamethasone valerate 0.1%	
generic	cream
Desonide 0.05%	
generic	oint
Desowen (Galderma)	
Fluocinolone acetonide 0.025%	
generic	cream

SOME TOPICAL DRUGS FOR ATOPIC DERMATITIS (continued)

Drug	Vehicle
Medium-Low Potency (continued)	
Flurandrenolide 0.05%	
Cordran (Aqua)	lotion
Cordran SP (Aqua)	cream
Fluticasone propionate 0.05%	
generic	cream
Cutivate (PharmaDerm)	
Hydrocortisone	
butyrate 0.1%	
generic	cream, oint, soln
Locoid (Triax)	cream, oint, soln
Locoid Lipocream (Triax)	cream
Hydrocortisone	
valerate 0.2%	
generic	cream
Prednicarbate 0.1% – generic	cream
Dermatop (Dermik)	
Triamcinolone	
acetonide 0.025%	
generic	oint
Triamcinolone	
acetonide 0.1%	
generic	lotion
Low Potency	
Alclometasone	
dipropionate 0.05%	
generic	cream, oint
Aclovate (GSK)	cream, oint
Betamethasone	
valerate 0.1%	
generic	lotion

Continued on next page.

SOME TOPICAL DRUGS FOR ATOPIC DERMATITIS (continued)

Drug	Vehicle
Low Potency (continued)	
Clocortolone 0.1%	
Cloderm (Valeant)	cream
Desonide 0.05%	
generic	cream, lotion
Desonate (Intendis)	gel
DesOwen (Galderma)	cream, lotion
Verdeso (Stiefel Labs)	foam
Fluocinolone acetonide 0.01%	
generic	cream, soln
Triamcinolone acetonide 0.025%	
generic	cream, lotion
Lowest Potency (may be ineffective for some indications)	
Hydrocortisone 0.5%[1]	
generic	cream, oint, lotion
Hydrocortisone 1.0%[1]	
generic	cream, oint, lotion
Hydrocortisone 2.5%	
generic	cream, oint, lotion

1. Available without a prescription.

widespread skin involvement who require long-term treatment. The risk of skin and other lymphomas also increases with the potency of the topical corticosteroids used and the duration of exposure.[21]

Topical Calcineurin Inhibitors – The topically applied calcineurin inhibitors tacrolimus and pimecrolimus are microbial-derived macrolides with a mechanism of action similar to that of cyclosporine (*Sandimmune*, and others). They can reduce itching and inflammation within a few days. Topical tacrolimus 0.1% is similar in efficacy to a topical corticosteroid with moderate potency and might be considered for long-term use in patients with topical corticosteroid-resistant atopic dermatitis, especially at sites such as the face or intertriginous areas where adverse effects from topical corticosteroid toxicity may be troublesome. Pimecrolimus is not as effective as a moderately potent topical corticosteroid, but it is an effective steroid-sparing therapy for mild to moderate atopic dermatitis.[22] Intermittent applications of 0.03% tacrolimus ointment 3 times weekly appear to increase the number of flare-free days and the time to relapse.[23]

Adverse effects, generally mild, include transient local itching, burning, stinging or erythema and a temporary increase in skin infections. Pimecrolimus is less likely than tacrolimus to cause these effects. These drugs do not cause cutaneous atrophy, and they can be used on the face, including areas around the mouth and eyes, and on the axillae and groin. Data are available showing that tacrolimus has been used safely in adults and children 2-15 years old for up to 4 years. In 2005, reports of malignancies in animals given large doses and of 8 skin malignancies and 12 lymphomas in adults and children treated with these drugs (not significantly higher than expected) prompted the FDA to issue a public health advisory about potential long-term risks of malignancy with topical tacrolimus and pimecrolimus. A retrospective cohort study found an increased risk of T-cell lymphoma among patients exposed to tacrolimus.[24] More long-term data are needed.[25]

Coal Tar – Coal tar preparations have anti-pruritic and anti-inflammatory effects, but they are messy and are now seldom recommended except in shampoo formulations. Adverse effects include skin irritation, folliculitis and photosensitivity.

Systemic Drugs – In many patients with atopic dermatitis, H_1-antihistamines are not very effective in relieving itching, probably because in addition to histamines, other mediators such as neuropeptides and cytokines also contribute to itching. Cetirizine, although not FDA-approved for this indication, was mildly effective and reduced the use of topical steroids in one 18-month study in infants with atopic dermatitis.[26]

Short courses of an oral corticosteroid such as prednisone may be needed in severe acute exacerbations of atopic dermatitis, but the drug should be tapered quickly, and intensified skin care with topical corticosteroids and calcineurin inhibitors should be started before tapering to reduce rebound inflammation. In patients with recalcitrant atopic dermatitis, cyclosporine and other immunomodulators have been used.

Anti-Infective Therapy – If a secondary infection with *Staphylococcus aureus* is present, a semi-synthetic penicillin or a first-generation cephalosporin such as cephalexin can be given for 7-10 days. Maintenance antibiotic treatment should be avoided because it may result in colonization by methicillin-resistant organisms. The topical anti-staphylococcal antibiotic mupirocin *(Bactroban)* applied three times daily to affected areas for 7-10 days may be effective. Twice-daily treatment for 5 days with a nasal preparation of mupirocin may reduce intranasal carriage of *S. aureus*.[27]

Nonpharmacologic Treatment – Skin hydration with application of moisturizers and emollients is important. Products containing ceramides such as *CeraVe* are reported to be more efficacious than traditional moisturizers.[28,29] Avoidance of irritating soaps, detergents or clothing, dust mites, extremes of temperature and humidity or anything else that triggers the itch/scratch cycle, plus trimming of fingernails, are all helpful in the management of atopic dermatitis. Identification and elimination of foods that exacerbate atopic dermatitis may sometimes also be helpful. Phototherapy has been effective in some patients. Allergen-specific immunotherapy is not recommended for treatment of atopic dermatitis.[20]

Drugs of Choice – Topical corticosteroid creams and ointments remain first-line choices for pharmacotherapy of atopic dermatitis. Pimecrolimus appears to be an effective steroid-sparing therapy for mild to moderate disease. Tacrolimus might be able to replace a potent corticosteroid for long-term treatment, especially on the face or intertriginous areas. Pimecrolimus generally costs slightly less than tacrolimus, but much more than generic topical corticosteroids.

URTICARIA

Acute urticaria is a self-limited condition that responds well to treatment with an H_1-antihistamine, preferably a second-generation drug such as cetirizine, fexofenadine, loratadine, desloratadine or levocetizirine.[30-32]

Chronic urticaria can last for months, years or even decades. Oral H_1-antihistamines decrease itching and reduce the number, size and duration of wheals. Taken regularly, they can prevent new wheals from appearing. Higher doses of a second-generation H_1-antihistamine are now recommended by some specialists for the treatment of chronic urticaria that does not respond to usual recommended doses.[33] First-generation sedating antihistamines such as diphenhydramine or hydroxyzine are still used for urticaria, but controlled trials are lacking.

The leukotriene receptor antagonist montelukast, alone or added to an H_1-antihistamine such as loratadine, has been effective against urticaria in some studies, but not in others. Topical corticosteroid creams and ointments are not effective in chronic urticaria. Short-term treatment with an oral corticosteroid or cyclosporine may be required in some patients.[34] Low doses of cyclosporine have been effective in patients with urticaria unresponsive to antihistamines.[35]

Patients should avoid nonspecific exacerbating factors for urticaria such as anything that raises body temperature. Patients with urticaria triggered by aspirin or other NSAIDs should not take these medications. Patients with known physical urticaria triggers such as cold, heat, light, or pressure should avoid them.[30]

The pathophysiologies of **urticarial vasculitis** and **nonallergic angio-edema,** including hereditary angioedema, are different from that of urticaria, and these diseases do not respond to conventional H_1-antihistamine treatment.[36]

ANAPHYLAXIS

Patients at risk for anaphylaxis should receive printed information about how to avoid confirmed relevant trigger factors, such as food or drugs. The Food Allergy and Anaphylaxis Network (www.foodallergy.org) provides support for patients with food allergies. If stinging insects are the trigger for anaphylaxis, patients should be referred to a specialist for venom immunotherapy, which provides long-lasting, potentially life-saving protection.[37]

All patients at risk of anaphylaxis should be equipped with epinephrine auto-injectors such as *EpiPen* or *Twinject*, which provide epinephrine in fixed doses of 0.15 mg and 0.3 mg. The recommended dose of epinephrine is 0.01 mg/kg intramuscularly (maximum 0.5 mg). Auto-injectors containing 0.15 mg are, therefore, optimal for young children weighing around 15 kg, and those containing 0.3 mg for children weighing 30 kg or more. Since no weight-appropriate dose for infants is available in an auto-injector, many physicians prescribe the 0.15 mg auto-injector (off-label) for this age group. Since no auto-injector provides an optimal dose for most children weighing between 15 and 30 kg, some physicians prescribe auto-injectors containing 0.3 mg epinephrine for children who have attained a weight of 22 or 23 kg.[38] Patients and caregivers need to be trained to use auto-injectors correctly and safely.[39]

Absorption of epinepherine after intramuscular injection is faster and the effect is less variable than after subcutaneous injection, but the needle lengths of *EpiPen* and *Twinject* may be too short for an intramuscular injection in some patients, including children.[40] After injection of epinephrine, patients should be taken to the nearest emergency department and observed after apparent recovery because, despite no further exposure to the trigger, anaphylaxis symptoms may recur within 72 hours in up to 20% of patients.[41] H_1-antihistamines are often used to treat anaphylaxis, but they do not prevent or relieve airway obstruction, hypotension or shock.

LARGE LOCAL ALLERGIC REACTIONS

Large local allergic reactions occurring, for example, at the sites of insect stings or bites appear within 24 hours. Although they may last for 5-7 days, they are self-limited. Local application of cold compresses and an oral second-generation H_1-antihistamine such as cetirizine may relieve itching. The H_1-antihistamine can be supplemented, if needed, with application of a topical corticosteroid cream to the skin for a few days. For severe large local reactions, oral prednisone 1 mg/kg, up to 50 mg daily for 5-7 days, should be prescribed. Venom immunotherapy can prevent anaphylactic and large local reactions to insect stings in patients who have had severe reactions and cannot avoid exposure to stinging insects.[42]

IMMUNOTHERAPY

Allergen-specific immunotherapy involving injection of gradually increasing doses of the causative allergen ("allergy shots") is effective in allergic rhinitis and allergic conjunctivitis (and in allergic asthma).[43,44] Standard subcutaneous allergen immunotherapy is limited by the potential for adverse effects, including anaphylaxis, and the requirement for regular (usually monthly) maintenance dosing for several years, but the benefits can persist for years after treatment is stopped. Insect venom immunotherapy is highly effective in preventing anaphylaxis triggered by stings from honeybees, yellow jackets, hornets and wasps.[45] Fire ant whole body extract immunotherapy can also protect against anaphylaxis. Sublingual immunotherapy for treatment of allergic rhinitis and allergic conjunctivitis due to airborne allergens is used in Europe and is currently being studied in the US and Canada. It appears to be effective.[46]

CONCLUSION

For treatment of **allergic rhinitis**, topical intranasal corticosteroids are the most effective drugs available. An oral second-generation H_1-antihistamine or an intranasal H_1-antihistamine is a good choice for mild to moderate symptoms. For **allergic conjunctivitis**, an oral second-generation H_1-antihistamine or a topical ophthalmic H_1-antihistamine/mast-cell stabilizer can be used. Allergen-specific immunotherapy is effective for both of these disorders, and the benefits can last for years after therapy is stopped.

In patients with **atopic dermatitis**, a topical corticosteroid with the lowest potency that relieves inflammation would be a cost-effective choice. The calcineurin inhibitors pimecrolimus *(Elidel)* and tacrolimus *(Protopic)* have the advantage over topical corticosteroids of not causing skin atrophy, adrenal suppression or ocular adverse effects, and are particularly useful on the face, but they are expensive and their long-term safety remains to be determined.

In acute and chronic **urticaria**, oral second-generation H_1-antihistamines are the most effective drugs for symptom relief. Topical corticosteroids are not effective.

Patients at **risk of anaphylaxis** recurrence should be equipped with epinephrine auto-injectors and taught when and how to use them.

1. Joint Task Force on Practice Parameters et al. The diagnosis and management of rhinitis: An updated practice parameter. J Allergy Clin Immunol 2008; 122:S1.
2. S Walker et al. Seasonal allergic rhinitis is associated with a detrimental effect on examination performance in United Kingdom teenagers: case-control study. J Allergy Clin Immunol 2007; 120:381.
3. FER Simons and KJ Simons. H_1-antihistamines. Current status and future directions. WAO Journal 2008; 1:145.
4. C Bachert. A review of the efficacy of desloratadine, fexofenadine, and levocetirizine in the treatment of nasal congestion in patients with allergic rhinitis. Clin Ther 2009; 31:921.
5. FER Simons on behalf of the Early Prevention of Asthma in Atopic Children (EPAAC) Study Group. Safety of levocetirizine treatment in young atopic children: an 18-month study. Pediatr Allergy Immunol 2007; 18:535.

6. MA Kaliner. Azelastine and olopatadine in the treatment of allergic rhinitis. Ann Allergy Asthma Immunol 2009; 103:373.
7. EO Meltzer et al. Comparative study of sensory attributes of two antihistamine nasal sprays: olopatadine 0.6% and azelastine 0.1%. Allergy and Asthma Proc 2008; 29:659.
8. C LaForce et al. Efficacy and safety of ciclesonide hydrofluoroalkane nasal aerosol once daily for the treatment of seasonal allergic rhinitis. Ann Allergy Asthma Immunol 2009; 103:166.
9. EO Meltzer et al. Efficacy and safety of once-daily fluticasone furoate nasal spray in children with seasonal allergic rhinitis treated for two weeks. Pediatr Allergy Immunol 2009; 20:279.
10. EO Meltzer et al. Preferences of adult patients with allergic rhinitis for the sensory attributes of fluticasone furoate versus fluticasone propionate nasal sprays: a randomized, multicenter, double-blind, single-dose, crossover study. Clin Ther 2008; 30:271.
11. PH Ratner et al. Mometasone furoate nasal spray is safe and effective for 1-year treatment of children with perennial allergic rhinitis. Int J Pediatr Otorhinolaryngol 2009; 73:651.
12. RC Hatton et al. Efficacy and safety of oral phenylephrine: systematic review and meta-analysis. Ann Pharmacother 2007; 41:381.
13. RF Lockey. Rhinitis medicamentosa and the stuffy nose. J Allergy Clin Immunol 2006; 118:1017.
14. Omalizumab (Xolair): an anti-IgE antibody for asthma. Med Lett Drugs Ther 2003; 45:67.
15. T Mainardi et al. Complementary and alternative medicine: herbs, phytochemicals and vitamins and their immunologic effects. J Allergy Clin Immunol 2009; 123:283.
16. E Schenkel. Oral antihistamines have proven efficacy in treating ocular symptoms of allergic rhinitis. J Allergy Clin Immunol 2007; 120:1473.
17. L Bielory and MH Friedlaender. Allergic conjunctivitis. Immunol Allergy Clin North Am 2008; 28:43.
18. V Yaylali et al. Comparative study of 0.1% olopatadine hydrochloride and 0.5% ketorolac tromethamine in the treatment of seasonal allergic conjunctivitis. Acta Ophthalmol Scand 2003; 81:378.
19. FM Baroody et al. Fluticasone furoate nasal spray reduces the nasal-ocular reflex: a mechanism for the efficacy of topical steroids in controlling allergic eye symptoms. J Allergy Clin Immunol 2009; 123:1342.
20. CA Akdis et al. Diagnosis and treatment of atopic dermatitis in children and adults: European Academy of Allergology and Clinical Immunology/American Academy of Allergy, Asthma and Immunology/PRACTALL Consensus Report. J Allergy Clin Immunol 2006; 118:152.
21. FM Arellano et al. Lymphoma among patients with atopic dermatitis and/or treated with topical immunosuppressants in the United Kingdom. J Allergy Clin Immunol 2009; 123:1111.
22. MMY El-Batawy et al. Topical calcineurin inhibitors in atopic dermatitis: a systematic review and meta-analysis. J Dermatol Sci 2009; 54:76.
23. D Breneman et al. Intermittent therapy for flare prevention and long-term disease control in stabilized atopic dermatitis: a randomized comparison of 3-times-weekly applications of tacrolimus ointment versus vehicle. J Am Acad Dermatol 2008; 58:990.

Drugs for Allergic Disorders

24. RL Hui et al. Association between exposure to topical tacrolimus or pimecrolimus and cancers. Ann Pharmacother 2009; 43:1956.
25. A Remitz and S Reitamo. Long-term safety of tacrolimus ointment in atopic dermatitis. Expert Opin Drug Saf 2009; 8:501.
26. TL Diepgen et al. Long-term treatment with cetirizine of infants with atopic dermatitis: a multi-country, double-blind, randomized, placebo-controlled trial (the ETAC trial) over 18 months. Pediatr Allergy Immunol 2002; 13:278.
27. JT Huang et al. Treatment of staphylococcus aureus colonization in atopic dermatitis decreases disease severity. Pediatrics 2009; 123:e808.
28. J Gupta et al. Intrinsically defective skin barrier function in children with atopic dermatitis correlates with disease severity. J Allergy Clin Immunol 2008; 121:725.
29. PC Anderson and JG Dinulos. Are the new moisturizers more effective? Curr Opin Pediatr 2009; 21:486.
30. RJ Powell et al. BSACI guidelines for the management of chronic urticaria and angio-oedema. Clin Exp Allergy 2007; 37:631.
31. FER Simons, on behalf of the Early Prevention of Asthma in Atopic Children (EPAAC) Study Group. H_1-antihistamine treatment in young atopic children: effect on urticaria. Ann Allergy Asthma Immunol 2007; 99:261.
32. JP Ortonne et al. Efficacy and safety of desloratadine in adults with chronic idiopathic urticaria: a randomized, double-blind, placebo-controlled, multicenter trial. Am J Clin Dermatol 2007; 8:37.
33. F Siebenhaar et al. High-dose desloratadine decreases wheal volume and improves cold provocation thresholds compared with standard-dose treatment in patients with acquired cold urticaria: a randomized, placebo-controlled, crossover study. J Allergy Clin Immunol 2009; 123:672.
34. M Morgan and DA Khan. Therapeutic alternatives for chronic urticaria: an evidence-based review, part 1. Ann Allergy Asthma Immunol 2008; 100:403.
35. D Doshi and MM Weinberger. Experience with cyclosporine in children with chronic idiopathic urticaria. Pediatr Dermatol 2009; 26:409.
36. BL Zuraw. Clinical practice. Hereditary angioedema. N Engl J Med 2008; 359:1027.
37. FER Simons. Anaphylaxis: recent advances in assessment and treatment. J Allergy Clin Immunol 2009; 124:625.
38. SF Kemp et al. Epinephrine: the drug of choice for anaphylaxis. A statement of the World Allergy Organization. Allergy 2008; 63:1061.
39. FER Simons et al. Hazards of unintentional injection of epinephrine from auto-injectors: a systematic review. Ann Allergy Asthma Immunol 2009; 102:282.
40. D Stecher et al. Epinephrine auto-injectors: is needle length adequate for delivery of epinephrine intramuscularly? Pediatrics 2009; 124:65.
41. KM Jarvinen et al. Use of multiple doses of epinephrine in food-induced anaphylaxis in children. J Allergy Clin Immunol 2008; 122:133.
42. DBK Golden et al. Venom immunotherapy reduces large local reactions to insect stings. J Allergy Clin Immunol 2009; 123:1371.
43. MA Calderon et al. Allergen injection immunotherapy for seasonal allergic rhinitis. Cochrane Database Syst Rev 2007; 1:CD001936.

44. HS Nelson. Multiallergen immunotherapy for allergic rhinitis and asthma. J Allergy Clin Immunol 2009; 123:763.
45. BM Bilo and F Bonifazi. Advances in Hymenoptera venom immunotherapy. Curr Opin Allergy Clin Immunol 2007; 7:567.
46. U Wahn et al. Efficacy and safety of 5-grass-pollen sublingual immunotherapy tablets in pediatric allergic rhinoconjunctivitis. J Allergy Clin Immunol 2009; 123:160.

FEXOFENADINE *(ALLEGRA)* AND FRUIT JUICE

Originally published in The Medical Letter – May 2011; 53:41

Fexofenadine (*Allegra,* and others) is the most recent second-generation H_1-antihistamine to become available over the counter (OTC). Cetirizine (*Zyrtec,* and others) and loratadine (*Claritin,* and others) are already available OTC. Cetirizine can be sedating in usual doses. Loratadine can be sedating in higher-than-usual doses. Fexofenadine remains nonsedating even in higher doses.[1]

The manufacturer of *Zyrtec* has responded to this new OTC product with television advertisements drawing attention to the label warning against taking fexofenadine with fruit juice. Many fruit juices such as grapefruit, orange and apple juice are organic anion transporting peptide (OATP) 1A2 inhibitors. OATP1A2 transporters are involved in the absorption of fexofenadine from the gastrointestinal tract. Inhibition of the activity of intestinal OATP1A2 reduces serum concentrations of fexofenadine by up to 70%, possibly reducing its effectiveness.[2] Patients can avoid this interaction by not drinking fruit juice within 4 hours before or 1-2 hours after taking fexofenadine.

1. Drugs for allergic disorders. Treat Guidel Med Lett 2010; 8:9.
2. DG Bailey. Fruit juice inhibition of uptake transport: a new type of food-drug interaction. Br J Clin Pharmacol 2010; 70:645.

Antithrombotic Drugs

Original publication date – October 2011 (revised March 2012)

Arterial thrombi are composed mainly of platelet aggregates held together by small amounts of fibrin. Antiplatelet drugs are the drugs of choice for prevention and treatment of arterial thrombosis, but anticoagulants are also effective, and their effects can add to those of antiplatelet drugs. Venous thrombi are composed mainly of fibrin and trapped red blood cells, with relatively few platelets. Anticoagulants are the agents of choice for prevention and treatment of venous thromboembolism and for prevention of cardioembolic events in patients with atrial fibrillation.

ANTIPLATELET DRUGS

Antiplatelet drugs are used mainly for primary and secondary prevention and treatment of acute coronary syndrome (ACS), which includes unstable angina/non-ST-elevation myocardial infarction (UA/NSTEMI), ST-elevation myocardial infarction (STEMI) and percutaneous coronary intervention (PCI).

ASPIRIN — Aspirin irreversibly acetylates cyclooxygenase-1, blocking thromboxane synthesis and inhibiting platelet activation and aggregation for the lifetime of the platelet (5-7 days). Its use slightly increases the risk of major bleeding. Aspirin can cause asthma and other hypersensitivity symptoms in aspirin-intolerant patients.

Antithrombotic Drugs

DRUGS OF CHOICE

Indication	Drugs
Primary Prevention	
Risk Factors	Aspirin
No Risk Factors	None[1]
Secondary Prevention	
Recent MI	Aspirin[2]
Ischemic Stroke	Aspirin $\pm$ dipyridamole; or clopidogrel
UA/NSTEMI	Aspirin
	$\pm$ clopidogrel or prasugrel or ticagrelor
	$\pm$ UFH or LMWH or fondaparinux[3]
	$\pm$ GPIIb/IIIa inhibitor
Acute MI (STEMI)	Aspirin
	+ clopidogrel or prasugrel or ticagrelor
	+ UFH or LMWH or fondaparinux[3]
	$\pm$ GPIIb/IIIa inhibitor
PCI	Aspirin
	+ clopidogrel or prasugrel or ticagrelor
	+ UFH or LMWH or bivalirudin
	$\pm$ GPIIb/IIIa inhibitor
VTE Treatment	LMWH or UFH or fondaparinux
	+ warfarin
VTE Prevention	
Hospitalized Medical Patients	Low-dose UFH, LMWH or fondaparinux
General Surgery	Low-dose UFH, LMWH or fondaparinux
Orthopedic Surgery	Fondaparinux or rivaroxaban or dabigatran[3] or LMWH or warfarin
Atrial Fibrillation	Aspirin[4] or warfarin or dabigatran or rivaroxaban[3] or apixaban[5]
Peripheral Arterial Disease	Aspirin[2]

UFH = Unfractionated heparin; LMWH = Low-molecular-weight heparin
1. Some clinicians offer aspirin to women >65 and men >45 years old.
2. Or, if intolerant to aspirin, clopidogrel.
3. Not FDA-approved for this indication.
4. For patients at low risk.
5. Not yet available in the US.

Aspirin prophylaxis reduces the incidence of MI and/or death by 15-25% in patients with UA/NSTEMI, STEMI or ischemic stroke, and in those undergoing PCI or a coronary artery bypass graft (CABG). Aspirin can also prevent MIs in asymptomatic men and ischemic stroke in asymptomatic women, but the risk-benefit ratio is less favorable because the thrombotic risk is lower and the benefit in preventing thrombosis is offset by a small increased risk of hemorrhagic stroke.[1,2]

DIPYRIDAMOLE — A pyrimidopyrimidine derivative, dipyridamole (*Persantine*, and others) inhibits platelet uptake of adenosine and blocks adenosine diphosphate (ADP)-induced platelet aggregation. It is also available in combination with aspirin (*Aggrenox*, and others).[3] Dipyridamole can cause severe headache and diarrhea, which tend to resolve with continued use.

A randomized, controlled trial (ESPRIT) in 2739 patients who had experienced a transient ischemic attack (TIA) or minor stroke in the previous 6 months found that a combination of extended-release dipyridamole (200 mg bid) and low-dose aspirin (30-325 mg per day) was more effective than aspirin alone in preventing a composite of vascular death, stroke, MI or major bleeding (173 vs. 216 events). However, more patients discontinued the combination (470 vs. 184), mainly because of headache.[4] The combination was not more effective than clopidogrel alone in preventing recurrent stroke.[5]

THIENOPYRIDINES — The thienopyridines ticlopidine (seldom used now because of its toxicity), clopidogrel *(Plavix)* and prasugrel *(Effient)* irreversibly inhibit P2Y12, a major ADP receptor on the platelet surface, increasing the risk of bleeding for the lifetime of the platelet (5-7 days). The delayed onset of action of these agents (they are prodrugs that must be metabolized to become active) can be problematic in patients who require a rapid antithrombotic effect.

Continued on page 38

DRUGS FOR ACUTE CORONARY SYNDROME

Drug	Usual Dosage
ANTIPLATELET DRUGS	
Aspirin – generic	75-81 mg PO daily
Dipyridamole (IR) – generic *Persantine* (Boehringer Ingelheim)	75-100 mg PO qid

Dipyridamole (ER)/aspirin[2] – generic
  Aggrenox (Boehringer Ingelheim)
	200 mg/25 mg PO bid
	  (morning and evening)

Clopidogrel – *Plavix* (Sanofi Aventis)	300-600 mg PO loading dose, 75 mg PO once daily
Prasugrel[3] – *Effient* (Lilly)	60 mg PO loading dose, 10 mg PO once daily[4]
Ticagrelor – *Brilinta* (AstraZeneca)	180 mg PO loading dose, 90 mg PO bid
Ticlopidine – generic	250 mg PO bid
GPIIb/IIIa INHIBITORS	

Abciximab – *ReoPro*
  (Centocor/Lilly)
	0.25 mg/kg bolus, then 0.125 mcg/kg/min
	  IV (max 10 mcg/min)

Eptifibatide – *Integrilin* (Merck)	180 mcg/kg bolus 1-2x (10 min apart), then 2 mcg/kg/min IV

Tirofiban – *Aggrastat* (Medicure)	0.4 mcg/kg/min x 30 min, then
	  0.1 mcg/kg/min IV
	PCI: 25 mcg/kg bolus over 3 min, then
	  0.1 mcg/kg/min IV[6,7]

ACT = Activated Coagulation Time
1. Irreversibility of antiplatelet drugs means that the effect persists for the lifetime of the platelet (5-7 days).
2. Should not be chewed or crushed.
3. Not recommended in patients >75 years-old, unless high risk, or in those with stroke or a history of TIA.

Renal Dosing	Reversibility of Antithrombotic Effect[1]
No dosage adjustment required; do not use if CrCl <10 mL/min	Irreversible, 50-100% dialyzable
No dosage adjustment required	Irreversible
No dosage adjustment required; do not use if CrCl <10 mL/min	Irreversible
No dosage adjustment required	Irreversible
No dosage adjustment required	Irreversible, not dialyzable
No dosage adjustment required	Reversible[5]
No dosage adjustment required	Irreversible
No dosage adjustment required	Not known
CrCl <50 mL/min: reduce maintenance dose to 1 mcg/kg/min	Irreversible, dialyzable
CrCl <30 mL/min: reduce dose by 50%	Irreversible, dialyzable

4. Reduce dose to 5 mg for patients <60 kg.
5. Recovery of platelet function after stopping the drug is about twice as rapid with ticagrelor as it is with clopidogrel.
6. Not an FDA-approved indication.
7. FG Kushner et al. Circulation 2009; 120:2271.

Continued on next page.

DRUGS FOR ACUTE CORONARY SYNDROME (continued)

Drug	Usual Dosage
ANTICOAGULANTS Unfractionated Heparin – generic	UA/NSTEMI: 60 units/kg bolus, then 12 units/kg/hr IV STEMI: 60 units/kg bolus, then 12 units/kg/hr IV PCI: 70-100 units/kg IV bolus, titrate to ACT 250-300 sec[8] (50-70 units/kg IV bolus if GP IIb/IIIa used, titrate to ACT 200-250 sec)
LOW-MOLECULAR-WEIGHT HEPARINS Enoxaparin – generic *Lovenox* (Sanofi Aventis)	UA/NSTEMI: 1 mg/kg SC q12h STEMI: 30 mg IV bolus plus 1 mg/kg SC, then 1 mg/kg SC q12h[9,10]
Dalteparin – *Fragmin* (Pfizer)	UA/NSTEMI: 120 IU/kg (max 10,000 IU) SC q12h
DIRECT THROMBIN INHIBITOR Bivalirudin – *Angiomax* (The Medicines Co.)	PCI: 0.75 mg/kg bolus then 1.75 mg/kg/h IV
FACTOR Xa INHIBITOR Fondaparinux[6] – generic *Arixtra* (GSK)	2.5 mg SC once daily[12,13]
VITAMIN K ANTAGONIST Warfarin – generic *Coumadin* (Bristol Myers Squibb)	2-10 mg PO daily[14]

8. With *Hemotec* device and 300-350 sec with *Hemochron* device.
9. Dose for patients <75 years old. For patients ≥75 years old, 0.75 mg/kg SC q12h.
10. For PCI, no additional dosing is needed if the last SC administration was <8 hrs before balloon inflation. If ≥8 hrs, an IV bolus of 0.3 mg/kg should be given.
11. Dose for patients <75 years old. For patients ≥75 years old, 1 mg/kg SC once daily

Renal Dosing	Reversibility of Antithrombotic Effect[1]
No dosage adjustment required	Protamine can reverse effects
CrCl <30 mL/min: UA/NSTEMI: 1 mg/kg SC once daily STEMI: 30 mg IV bolus plus 1mg/kg SC, then 1 mg/kg SC once daily[11]	Protamine (~60% neutralized)
CrCl <30 mL/min: based on anti-Xa levels	Protamine (~60% neutralized)
CrCl <30 mL/min: decrease infusion to 1mg/kg/h	No antidote, dialyzable
CrCl <30 mL/min: do not use	No antidote, dialyzable
No dosage adjustment required[15]	Vitamin K

12. Oasis – 6 Trial Group. JAMA 2006; 295:1519.
13. For STEMI, initial dose is given IV.
14. Monitor daily and adjust dose until results in therapeutic range (INR 2-3) for >24 hrs. Dose will vary based on INR.
15. Patients with renal failure may have an increased risk of bleeding.

Ticlopidine can cause skin reactions, cytopenias and thrombotic thrombocytopenic purpura; it has largely been replaced by clopidogrel.

Patient response to **clopidogrel** is variable. Whether those who are poor metabolizers of clopidogrel have a higher incidence of cardiovascular events is controversial.[6] Some clinicians recommend pharmacogenetic testing for CYP450 polymorphisms before prescribing a long course of clopidogrel.[7] Proton pump inhibitors, particularly omeprazole (*Prilosec*, and others), inhibit CYP2C19 and can interfere with activation of clopidogrel, but the results of some studies suggest that they do not increase adverse cardiovascular outcomes.[8]

Prasugrel appears to be more effective than clopidogrel, but is associated with a greater risk of bleeding.[9] Prasugrel is not recommended for patients with a history of stroke or TIA, or those $\geq$75 years old unless they are at high risk (diabetes or prior MI); the risk of bleeding is greater in older patients, and the benefit is less clear.

TICAGRELOR — Ticagrelor (*Brilinta*) binds reversibly to the same P2Y12 receptor as the thienopyridines. In one study (PLATO), ticagrelor plus aspirin was more effective than clopidogrel plus aspirin in preventing cardiovascular death, with no increase in overall major bleeding. Ticagrelor was, however, associated with an increase in non-CABG-related bleeding and a trend toward a higher risk of hemorrhagic stroke.[10] A subgroup analysis of the PLATO results showed that ticagrelor was not superior to clopidogrel in the subset of patients in North America, possibly due to use of higher doses of aspirin in the US. The US labeling of the drug, therefore, includes a boxed warning against using >100 mg of aspirin per day.[11]

GLYCOPROTEIN IIb/IIIa (GPIIb/IIIa) RECEPTOR ANTAGONISTS — The GPIIb/IIIa receptor antagonists, which are administered intravenously, prevent platelet aggregation by competing with fibrinogen and von Willebrand factor for platelet receptors.

Abciximab *(ReoPro)* is the Fab fragment of a chimeric monoclonal anti-body to the GPIIb/IIIa receptor that binds to both activated and non-activated platelets. While the plasma half-life of abciximab is only 30 minutes, its strong affinity for platelets results in measurable platelet inhibition for 24-48 hours, with low levels still detectable after 15 days. **Eptifibatide** *(Integrilin)* and **tirofiban** *(Aggrastat)* bind reversibly to the GPIIb/IIIa receptor of activated platelets. Bleeding at arterial access sites is the most common complication of these drugs. GPIIb/IIIa inhibitors, particularly abciximab, can also cause profound acute thrombocytopenia.

PARENTERAL ANTICOAGULANTS

HEPARIN — Heparins act by combining with plasma antithrombin to form a complex that is more active than antithrombin alone in neutraliz-ing thrombin and factor Xa. Unfractionated heparin (UFH) has numerous disadvantages compared to low-molecular-weight heparin (LMWH): it is more likely to cause heparin-induced thrombocytopenia and has a more variable anticoagulant response that requires monitoring. It also has advantages over LMWH, however, that have kept it from becoming obso-lete: its anticoagulant effect can be more rapidly reversed and more completely neutralized by protamine; it is not cleared by the kidneys and therefore may be safer in patients with renal insufficiency; and it directly inhibits the contact activation pathway that is important in the genesis of thrombi in stents, filters and catheter tips.

LMWH — LMWHs, produced by cleaving UFH into shorter chains, inhibit factor Xa more than they inhibit thrombin. Compared to UFH, LMWHs have longer half-lives that permit fewer doses per day, and their greater bioavailability leads to a more predictable anticoagulant response. In clinical trials comparing them with UFH, they have generally been at least as effective and as safe. Three LMWHs, enoxaparin (*Lovenox*, and others), dalteparin *(Fragmin)* and tinzaparin *(Innohep)*, have been approved by the FDA; they generally appear to be similar, but in clinical trials in patients with UA/NSTEMI, enoxaparin has been associated with

DRUGS FOR VENOUS THROMBOEMBOLISM

Drug	Dosage for Treatment
ANTICOAGULANTS	
Unfractionated Heparin	Initial: 80 units/kg IV bolus then 18 units/kg/hr or 250 units/kg SC^2 then 250 units/kg q12h
LOW-MOLECULAR-WEIGHT HEPARINS	
Enoxaparin[3]	1 mg/kg SC bid or 1.5 mg/kg once daily
Dalteparin[3]	100 IU/kg SC bid[4] or 200 IU/kg once daily[5]
Tinzaparin[3]	175 IU/kg SC once daily
VITAMIN K ANTAGONIST	
Warfarin	2-10 mg PO once daily[6]
DIRECT THROMBIN INHIBITORS	
Dabigatran[3]	150 mg PO bid[4,7]
Desirudin[3]	No data
FACTOR Xa INHIBITORS	
Fondaparinux[3]	5-10 mg SC^{10} once daily
Rivaroxaban[3]	15 mg PO bid for 3 weeks, then 20 mg once daily[4,12]
Apixaban[13]	5-10 mg PO bid or 20 mg PO daily[14]

1. For elective hip or knee arthroplasty, prophylaxis is recommended for a minimum of 10 days after surgery, and for hip arthroplasty, up to 35 days (WH Geerts et al. Chest 2008; 133:3815).
2. Initial dose is 333 units/kg for unmonitored dosing regimen.
3. Dosage adjustments may be necessary in renal insufficiency.
4. Dose only FDA-approved for this indication.
5. FDA-approved dose for cancer patients x 30 days, then 150 IU/kg SC daily x 5 months (not to exceed 18,000 IU/day).
6. Monitor daily and adjust dose until results in therapeutic range (INR 2-3) for $\geq$24 hours.
7. S Schulman et al. N Engl J Med 2009; 361:1342.

better outcomes than dalteparin or tinzaparin. Enoxaparin has been at least as safe as UFH in patients undergoing elective PCI.[12]

LMWHs are often used to treat or prevent venous thromboembolism (VTE). For initial treatment of deep vein thrombosis (DVT), LMWH is generally preferred to UFH. In a controlled trial in an ICU (PROTECT), dalteparin was not superior to UFH in preventing DVT, the primary

Dosage for Prophylaxis[1]

5000 units SC q 8-12h

30 mg SC bid or 40 mg SC once daily
2500-5000 IU SC once daily
75 IU/kg SC[4]

2-10 mg PO once daily[6]

150 mg PO bid[4,8]
15 mg SC q12h[9]

2.5 mg SC once daily[11]
10 mg PO once daily
2.5 mg PO bid[15]

8. A dose of 220 mg (two 110-mg capsules) once daily is approved for VTE prophylaxis in Canada.
9. Use of desirudin has only been studied for up to 12 days.
10. 5 mg if <50 kg, 7.5 mg if 50-100 kg, 10 mg if >100 kg.
11. Dose for adults ≥50 kg. Contraindicated for patients weighing <50 kg.
12. EINSTEIN Investigators. N Engl J Med 2010; 363:2499.
13. Not yet available in the US.
14. Botticelli Investigators Writing Committee. J Thromb Haemost 2008; 6:1313.
15. MR Lassen et al. Lancet 2010; 375:807.

endpoint, but dalteparin-treated patients had significantly fewer pulmonary emboli.[13]

FONDAPARINUX — Fondaparinux (*Arixtra*, and others), a synthetic analog of the pentasaccharide sequence of heparin, binds antithrombin with high affinity and inhibits factor Xa indirectly through antithrombin without neutralizing thrombin. The drug has a long half-life and requires injection only once daily. Fondaparinux accumulates in patients with renal insufficiency, which can be problematic in the elderly, and is contraindicated in patients with a CrCl <30 mL/min.

Fondaparinux appears to be as effective and safe as UFH or LMWH for prophylaxis and treatment of VTE and much less likely to cause heparin-induced thrombocytopenia.[14,15] It may also be used as an alternative to UFH or LMWH in UA/NSTEMI or STEMI.[12] In patients who underwent PCI, however, fondaparinux provided no added benefit and was associated with more catheter thrombosis.[16,17]

DIRECT THROMBIN INHIBITORS — Unlike heparins and fondaparinux, direct thrombin inhibitors inhibit clot-bound as well as circulating thrombin.

Bivalirudin *(Angiomax)*, which is given IV and has a short half-life, can be used instead of heparin in patients undergoing PCI; in one controlled trial, it significantly reduced the incidence of major bleeding compared to unfractionated heparin, but it did not provide a net benefit in outcomes.[18] In another study, however, in patients with STEMI undergoing primary PCI, use of bivalirudin alone resulted in lower death rates and less major bleeding than heparin plus a GPIIb/IIIa inhibitor.[19]

Desirudin *(Iprivask)* is a hirudin analog approved by the FDA for prevention of VTE after hip arthroplasty. It appears to be more effective than enoxaparin in preventing DVT after elective hip arthroplasty, but it must be injected twice daily and can cause life-threatening allergic reactions.[20]

ORAL ANTICOAGULANTS

WARFARIN (*Coumadin*, and others) — Vitamin K antagonists such as warfarin, which require monitoring, were for a long time the only oral anticoagulants available. Anticoagulation with warfarin reduces the risk of thromboembolic stroke in patients with atrial fibrillation by 60% or

DRUGS FOR ATRIAL FIBRILLATION

Drug	Dosage
Aspirin[1]	75-81 mg PO daily
Warfarin	2-10 mg PO daily[2]
Rivaroxaban	20 mg PO daily[3-5]
Dabigatran	150 mg PO bid[4]
Apixaban[6]	5 mg PO bid[7]

1. For patients at low risk.
2. Monitor daily until results in therapeutic range (INR 2-3) for >24 hrs.
3. Not FDA-approved for this indication.
4. Dosage adjustments may be necessary in renal insufficiency.
5. MR Patel et al. N Engl J Med 2011, Aug 10 (epub).
6. Not yet available in the US.
7. CB Granger et al. N Engl J Med 2011, Aug 28 (epub).

more and is more effective for this indication than antiplatelet therapy. With an annual rate of major bleeding of about 1-2% and an absolute increase in the rate of intracranial hemorrhage of about 0.2%, the benefits of warfarin far surpass the risks. The main drawback of warfarin is the variability in dosage requirements and the need for close monitoring to keep the international normalized ratio (INR) in the therapeutic range. Recently, 3 new oral anticoagulants that do not require monitoring have achieved good results in clinical trials.[21]

DABIGATRAN *(Pradaxa)* — In a randomized trial (RE-LY), fixed doses of the oral direct thrombin inhibitor dabigatran were at least as effective and safe as adjusted-dose warfarin in patients with atrial fibrillation followed for a median of 2 years.[22] For treatment of acute VTE, fixed-dose dabigatran was also as effective as adjusted-dose warfarin in preventing recurrent VTE, and as safe.[23] Unlike warfarin, however, the anticoagulant effect of dabigatran is irreversible, which is problematic if bleeding occurs or emergency surgery is needed. It also must be taken twice daily, a potential disadvantage for compliance with long-term use.

RIVAROXABAN *(Xarelto)* — In one study, the oral direct factor Xa inhibitor rivaroxaban was non-inferior to enoxaparin followed by warfarin for acute and continued treatment of VTE, with no increase in major bleeding.[24] It is approved by the FDA for prophylactic use after knee or hip replacement and for prevention of stroke and systemic embolism in patients with non-valvular atrial fibrillation (20 mg once daily). Rivaroxaban was more effective than enoxaparin for prophylactic use after knee or hip replacement, with no significant increase in bleeding.[25] In another trial (ROCKET AF), it was non-inferior to warfarin for prevention of stroke or systemic embolism in patients with non-valvular atrial fibrillation.[26,27] Rivaroxaban requires no monitoring and is taken once daily.

APIXABAN *(Eliquis)* — Another factor Xa inhibitor, apixaban, which has not yet been approved by the FDA for any indication, was more effective than warfarin in a randomized trial (ARISTOTLE) in preventing stroke or systemic embolism in patients with atrial fibrillation, with a lower rate of major bleeding.[28] In 2 other randomized controlled trials, apixaban was more effective than once-daily enoxaparin in preventing VTE after knee or hip replacement, without causing an increase in bleeding.[29,30] In high-risk patients after an acute coronary syndrome, however, addition of apixaban to antiplatelet therapy increased major bleeding and did not provide any benefit.[31]

1. Aspirin for the prevention of cardiovascular disease: U.S. Preventive Services Task Force recommendation statement. Ann Intern Med 2009; 150:396.
2. Antithrombotic Trialists' (ATT) Collaboration. Aspirin in the primary and secondary prevention of vascular disease: collaborative meta-analysis of individual participant data from randomised trials. Lancet 2009; 373:1849.
3. Aggrenox – A combination of antiplatelet drugs for stroke prevention. Med Lett Drugs Ther 2000; 42:11.
4. ESPRIT Study Group. Aspirin plus dipyridamole versus aspirin alone after cerebral ischaemia of arterial origin (ESPRIT): randomised controlled trial. Lancet 2006; 367:1665.
5. RL Sacco et al. Aspirin and extended-release dipyridamole versus clopidogrel for recurrent stroke. N Engl J Med 2008; 359:1238.
6. DM Roden and AR Shuldiner. Responding to the clopidogrel warning by the US Food and Drug Administration: real life is complicated. Circulation 2010; 122:445.

7. L Wang et al. Genomics and drug response. N Engl J Med 2011; 364:1144.
8. Drugs for treatment of peptic ulcer disease and GERD. Treat Guidel Med Lett 2011; 9:55.
9. Prasugrel (Effient) vs. clopidogrel (Plavix). Med Lett Drugs Ther 2009; 51:69.
10. L Wallentin et al. Ticagrelor versus clopidogrel in patients with acute coronary syndromes. N Engl J Med 2009; 361:1045.
11. Ticagrelor (Brilinta) – better than clopidogrel (Plavix)? Med Lett Drugs Ther 2011; 53:69.
12. RS Wright et al. 2011 ACCF/AHA focused update of the guidelines for the management of patients with unstable angina/non-ST-elevation myocardial infarction (updating the 2007 guideline). J Am Coll Cardiol 2011; 57:1920.
13. PROTECT Investigators. Dalteparin versus unfractionated heparin in critically ill patients. N Engl J Med 2011; 364:1305.
14. WH Geerts et al. Prevention of venous thromboembolism: American College of Chest Physicians evidence-based clinical practice guidelines (8th edition). Chest 2008; 133:381s.
15. TE Warkentin et al. Prevalence and risk of preexisting heparin-induced thrombocytopenia antibodies in patients with acute VTE. Chest 2011; 140:366.
16. The Oasis-6 Trial Group. Effects of fondaparinux on mortality and reinfarction in patients with acute ST-segment elevation myocardial infarction: the OASIS-6 randomized trial. JAMA 2006; 295:1519.
17. RM Califf. Fondaparinux in ST-segment elevation myocardial infarction: the drug, the strategy, the environment or all of the above? JAMA 2006; 295:1579.
18. A Kastrati et al. Bivalirudin versus unfractionated heparin during percutaneous coronary intervention. N Engl J Med 2008; 359:688.
19. GW Stone et al. Bivalirudin during primary PCI in acute myocardial infarction. N Engl J Med 2008; 358:2218.
20. Desirudin (Iprivask) for DVT prevention. Med Lett Drugs Ther 2010; 52:85.
21. JW Eikelboom and JI Weitz. New anticoagulants. Circulation 2010; 121:1523.
22. Dabigatran etexilate (Pradaxa) - a new oral anticoagulant. Med Lett Drugs Ther 2010; 52:89.
23. S Schulman et al. Dabigatran versus warfarin in the treatment of acute venous thromboembolism. N Engl J Med 2009; 361:2342.
24. EINSTEIN Investigators. Oral rivaroxaban for symptomatic venous thromboembolism. N Engl J Med 2010; 363:2499.
25. AG Turpie et al. Rivaroxaban for the prevention of venous thromboembolism after hip or knee arthroplasty. Pooled analysis of four studies. Thromb Haemost 2011; 105:444.
26. MR Patel et al. Rivaroxaban versus warfarin in nonvalvular atrial fibrillation. N Engl J Med 2011; 365:883.
27. Rivaroxaban (Xarelto) – a new oral anticoagulant. Med Lett Drugs Ther 2011; 53:65.
28. CB Granger et al. Apixaban versus warfarin in patients with atrial fibrillation. N Engl J Med 2011 Aug 27 (epub).
29. MR Lassen et al. Apixaban versus enoxaparin for thromboprophylaxis after knee replacement (ADVANCE-2): a randomized double-blind trial. Lancet 2010; 375:807.
30. MR Lassen et al. Apixaban versus enoxaparin for thromboprophylaxis after hip replacement. N Engl J Med 2010; 363:2487.
31. JH Alexander et al. Apixaban with antiplatelet therapy after acute coronary syndrome. N Engl J Med 2011 Jul 24 (epub).

PROTHROMBIN COMPLEX CONCENTRATES TO REVERSE WARFARIN-RELATED BLEEDING

Originally published in The Medical Letter – October 2011; 53:78

Warfarin-related bleeding, especially intracranial hemorrhage, can be catastrophic. Several products are available to reverse warfarin's anticoagulant effect.[1]

VITAMIN K — The vitamin K-dependent coagulation factors are II, VII, IX and X. Administration of vitamin K can take more than 24 hours to fully restore these factors. In patients with serious or life-threatening warfarin-

SOME PROTHROMBIN COMPLEX CONCENTRATES*

Product	Composition	
PROTHROMBIN COMPLEX CONCENTRATE (PCC) – 3 FACTORS		
Factor IX Complex (*Profilnine SD* – Grifols)[1,2]	Factor II: <150 units Factor VII: ≤35 units	Factor IX: 100 units Factor X: ≤100 units
Factor IX Complex (*Bebulin* – Baxter)[2,3]	Factor II: 24-38 units/mL Factor VII: 0.05-0.20 units[4]	Factor IX: 200-1200 units[5] Factor X: 24-38 units/mL
PROTHROMBIN COMPLEX CONCENTRATE (PCC) – 4 FACTORS		
Prothromplex Total 600 IU (Baxter)[3,6]	Factor II: 20-45 units/mL Factor VII: 25 units/mL	Factor IX: 30 units/mL Factor X: 30 units/mL
Beriplex P/N (CSL Behring)[3,6,7]	Factor II: 20-48 units/mL Factor VII: 10-25 units/mL	Factor IX: 20-31 units/mL Factor X: 22-60 units/mL
Octaplex (Octapharma)[3,6,7]	Factor II: 11-38 units/mL Factor VII: 9-24 units/mL	Factor IX: 25 units/mL Factor X: 18-30 units/mL
Cofact (Sanquin)[6,7]	Factor II: 14-35 units/mL Factor VII: 7-20 units/mL	Factor IX: 25 units/mL Factor X: 14-35 units/mL

*Non-activated. Activated PCCs are associated with an increased risk of thromboembolic events.
1. Factor units per 100 factor IX units
2. Only FDA-approved for factor IX deficiency due to hemophilia.
3. Also contains heparin.
4. Factor units per 1 factor IX unit.

related bleeding, vitamin K is usually given IV in a dose of 10 mg over about 30 minutes (to reduce the risk of anaphylaxis), and fresh-frozen plasma, recombinant factor VIIa or prothrombin complex concentrate (PCC) may be given in addition.[2]

FRESH-FROZEN PLASMA — The plasma product most likely to be available in emergency departments to rapidly replace vitamin K-dependent clotting factors is fresh-frozen plasma (FFP). When the speed of replacement is critical, however, as in warfarin-associated intracranial hemorrhage, FFP has some drawbacks: it requires blood typing and thawing, which can take 90 minutes or more, requires infusion of large volumes

Dose	Availability in US
Based on desired increased in plasma factor IX	Yes
Based on desired increase in plasma factor IX	Yes
Based on desired INR of 1.0	No (only in Austria)
25-50 IU/kg (factor IX); not to exceed 3 IU/kg/min	No (only in Europe and Canada[8])
25-50 IU/kg (factor IX); based on desired INR $\leq$2.1	No (only in Europe and Canada[8])
Based on desired INR $\leq$2.1	No (only in Europe)

5. Factor units per 20 mL vial.
6. Also contains proteins.
7. Also contains sodium.
8. From Canadian Blood Sources.

of fluid which can overload elderly patients and those with heart disease, and rarely can cause transfusion-related acute lung injury.

RECOMBINANT FACTOR VIIa — Recombinant factor VIIa has been used off-label to treat warfarin-associated intracranial hemorrhage.[3] It has been successful in stopping hemorrhage in some patients,[4] but its use has been associated with an increased risk of stroke and systemic embolus, and its effect on patient outcomes compared to PCC remains to be established.

PROTHROMBIN COMPLEX CONCENTRATES — A number of studies have shown that PCC can lower INR more rapidly than FFP.[5] US, British and French guidelines for reversal of warfarin-related bleeding recommend PCC as the treatment of choice to accompany vitamin K. The best evidence for the superior effectiveness of PCC in stopping bleeding coupled with a low incidence of thrombotic events is with 4-factor products.[6]

The composition of PCC products is variable. Those available in the US include clotting factors II, IX and X, but only small amounts of factor VII (3-factor PCC). Some clinicians, therefore, also give FFP to replace factor VII when using a 3-factor PCC to reverse warfarin-related bleeding. Products available outside the US contain a significant amount of factor VII as well (4-factor PCC).

CONCLUSION — Prothrombin complex concentrate could be helpful in reversing life-threatening warfarin-related bleeding.

1. LT Goodnough and A Shander. How I treat warfarin-associated coagulopathy in patients with intracerebral hemorrhage. Blood 2011; 117:6091.
2. J Ansell et al. Pharmacology and management of the vitamin K antagonists: American College of Chest Physicians Evidence-Based Clinical Practice Guidelines (8th Edition). Chest 2008; 133:160S.
3. MT Robinson et al. Safety of recombinant activated factor VII in patients with warfarin-associated hemorrhages of the central nervous system. Stroke 2010; 41:1459.
4. WD Freeman et al. Recombinant factor VIIa for rapid reversal of warfarin anticoagulation in acute intracranial hemorrhage. Mayo Clin Proc 2004; 79: 1495.

5. EM Bershad and JI Suarez. Prothrombin complex concentrates for oral anticoagulant therapy-related intracranial hemorrhage: a review of the literature. Neurocrit Care 2010; 12:403.
6. KS Schick et al. Prothrombin complex concentrate in surgical patients: retrospective evaluation of vitamin K antagonist reversal and treatment of severe bleeding. Crit Care 2009; 13:R191.

DRUGS FOR
Asthma

Original publication date – February 2012

RECOMMENDATIONS: Use of a short-acting bronchodilator as needed for relief of symptoms may be sufficient for asthma patients whose symptoms are infrequent, mild and transient. In patients with more frequent or more severe cough, wheeze, chest tightness or shortness of breath, regular use of a controller medication is recommended. Low daily doses of an inhaled corticosteroid suppress airway inflammation and reduce the risk of exacerbations. Higher inhaled corticosteroid doses may be needed in patients with more severe disease. In patients who remain symptomatic despite compliance with inhaled corticosteroid treatment and good inhalational technique, addition of a long-acting beta-2 agonist is recommended. In patients ≥12 years old with uncontrolled allergic asthma, omalizumab can be added. For patients of any age with allergic asthma, allergen immunotherapy may provide long-lasting benefits.

Failure of pharmacologic treatment can usually be attributed to lack of adherence to prescribed medications, uncontrolled co-morbid conditions, or continued exposure to tobacco smoke or other airborne pollutants, allergens or irritants.

INHALATION DEVICES

Inhalation is the preferred route of delivery for most asthma drugs. Chlorofluorocarbons (CFCs), which have ozone-depleting properties, are being phased out as propellants in metered-dose inhalers. Non-chlorinated hydrofluoroalkane (HFA) propellants, which do not deplete the ozone layer, are being used instead.

Metered-dose inhalers (MDIs) require coordination of inhalation with hand-actuation of the device. Valved holding chambers (VHCs) or spacers can help young children or elderly patients use MDIs effectively. VHCs have one-way valves that prevent the patient from exhaling into the device, eliminating the need for coordinated actuation and inhalation. Spacers are open tubes placed on the mouthpiece of an MDI. Both VHCs and spacers retain the large particles emitted from the MDI, preventing their deposition in the oropharynx and leading to a higher proportion of small respirable particles being inhaled.

Dry powder inhalers (DPIs), which are breath-actuated, can be used in patients who are capable of performing a rapid deep inhalation.

Delivery of inhaled asthma medications through a **nebulizer** with a face mask or mouthpiece is less dependent on the patient's coordination and cooperation, but more time-consuming than delivery through an MDI or DPI.

SHORT-ACTING BETA-2 AGONISTS

Inhaled short-acting beta-2 agonists (SABAs), such as albuterol, are used for rapid relief of asthma symptoms. Their onset of action occurs within 5 minutes; their peak effect occurs within 30-60 minutes and they have a duration of action of 4-6 hours.[1] SABAs do not decrease the inflammation of the airways that occurs in asthma. They should only be used as needed for relief of symptoms or for prevention of exercise-induced bronchoconstriction (EIB). In patients whose asthma is under control, SABAs should be needed infrequently ($\leq$2 days/week).[2]

Adverse Effects – Inhaled SABAs can cause tachycardia, QTc interval prolongation, tremor, anxiety, hyperglycemia, hypokalemia and hypo-magnesemia, especially if used in high doses. Tolerance (some loss of effectiveness) can occur with daily use.[3]

CORTICOSTEROIDS

Inhaled – In all age groups with persistent asthma, whether it is mild, moderate or severe, inhaled corticosteroids (ICSs) are the most effective long-term treatment for control of symptoms. In randomized controlled trials, they have been significantly more effective than long-acting beta-2 agonists, leukotriene modifiers, cromolyn or theophylline in improving pulmonary function, preventing symptoms and exacerbations, reducing the need for emergency department treatment, and decreasing deaths due to asthma.[4] ICSs are most effective when used daily, and their efficacy does not persist after they are stopped.[5]

Most of the beneficial effects of ICSs are achieved at relatively low doses. The ideal dose for a given patient is the lowest dose that maintains asthma control; this dose may change seasonally and over time. Current evidence suggests that, at usual doses, all ICSs are similar in efficacy and safety; they are not interchangeable on a per-microgram or per-puff basis because the dose varies with the drug, the formulation and the delivery device.[6]

Adverse Effects – Local adverse effects of ICSs may include oral can-didiasis (thrush), dysphonia, and reflex cough and bronchospasm. Their incidence can be reduced by use of a valved holding chamber (VHC) or a spacer, and by mouth-rinsing after inhalation.

Clinically relevant adverse effects on hypothalamic-pituitary-adrenal (HPA) axis function generally do not occur with low- or medium-dose

ICSs. Regular administration of low- or medium-dose ICSs may reduce growth velocity slightly during the first year of treatment, but final adult height does not appear to be affected.[7] Patients who require high-dose ICS treatment should be monitored for HPA axis suppression, changes in bone density, and development of cataracts or glaucoma. ICSs do not increase the risk of pneumonia in patients with asthma.[8]

Oral – Oral systemic glucocorticoids are the most effective drugs available for exacerbations of asthma incompletely responsive to bronchodilators. Even when an acute exacerbation responds to bronchodilators, addition of a short course of an oral glucocorticoid can decrease symptoms and may prevent a relapse. For asthma exacerbations, daily systemic gluco-corticoids are generally required for only 3-10 days, after which no tapering is needed.

Oral glucocorticoids should only rarely be used as long-term control medications and then only in that small minority of patients with uncon-trolled severe persistent asthma. In this situation, an oral glucocorticoid should be given at the lowest effective dose, preferably on alternate mornings, in order to produce the least toxicity.

LONG-ACTING BETA-2 AGONISTS

Monotherapy with an inhaled long-acting beta-2 agonist (LABA), such as salmeterol or formoterol, is not recommended. If a LABA is required, it should be used in combination with an ICS, preferably in the same inhaler. The combination inhalers salmeterol/fluticasone *(Advair)*, for-moterol/budesonide *(Symbicort)* and formoterol/mometasone *(Dulera)* are FDA-approved for use in patients with persistent asthma that is not well-controlled on an ICS alone. The addition of a LABA improves lung function, decreases symptoms and exacerbations, and reduces rescue use of short-acting beta-2 agonists.[9,10]

TREATMENT OF ASTHMA

Asthma Severity	Recommended Regimen[1]
MILD INTERMITTENT	SABA as needed
MILD PERSISTENT	
Preferred	Low-dose ICS[2]
Alternatives	Montelukast (or zafirlukast) or theophylline
MODERATE PERSISTENT	
Preferred	Low-dose ICS[2] + a LABA[3]
Alternatives	Medium-dose ICS[2] OR Low-dose ICS[2] + a leukotriene modifier or theophylline
SEVERE PERSISTENT	
Preferred	Medium- or high-dose ICS[2] + a LABA[3,4]
Alternatives	Medium-dose ICS[2] + a leukotriene modifier or theophylline

SABA = inhaled short-acting beta-2 agonist; ICS = inhaled corticosteroid; LABA = inhaled long-acting beta-2 agonist
1. For patients ≥12 years old. Treatment should be adjusted based on response.
2. The ideal dose of an ICS is the lowest dose that maintains asthma control.
3. The FDA recommends stopping a LABA once symptoms are controlled.
4. In patients who remain uncontrolled despite aggressive treatment with a high-dose ICS plus a LABA, oral glucocorticoids are sometimes added. Addition of omalizumab can be considered in patients with allergic asthma.

Adverse Effects – LABAs, especially if used in higher-than-recommended doses, can cause tremor, muscle cramps, tachycardia and other cardiac effects. Tolerance (some loss of efficacy) can occur with daily use of a LABA.[3]

An FDA meta-analysis found that use of a LABA was associated with an increased risk of asthma-related hospitalization, intubation and death; the greatest risk was in children 4-11 years old. These results prompted the FDA to recommend that LABAs be discontinued once asthma is controlled. A secondary analysis of the original meta-analysis did not find a significant increase in risk in a subset of patients who were assigned to use an ICS with a LABA.[11] The manufacturers of LABAs are conducting post-marketing trials to assess the safety of a LABA-ICS combination compared to that of an ICS alone.[12]

LEUKOTRIENE MODIFIERS

Leukotriene modifiers are less-effective alternatives to low-dose ICS treatment for patients who are unable or unwilling to use an ICS.[13] They are also generally less effective than an inhaled LABA as add-on therapy for patients not well controlled on an ICS alone. In one small study, some children with asthma uncontrolled on an ICS demonstrated a better response to step-up treatment with a leukotriene modifier than with a LABA.[10]

Adverse Effects – Montelukast is considered safe for long-term use. Both zafirlukast and (especially) zileuton have been reported to cause life-threatening hepatic injury; liver function tests should be monitored and patients should be warned to discontinue the medication immediately if abdominal pain, nausea, jaundice, itching or lethargy occur. Rarely, Churg-Strauss vasculitis has been reported with montelukast and zafirlukast; in most cases, this was likely a consequence of corticosteroid withdrawal rather than a direct effect of the drug.[13] The FDA has received post-marketing reports of psychiatric symptoms, including suicidality, with leukotriene modifiers.

ANTICHOLINERGICS

Ipratropium bromide is an inhaled short-acting anticholinergic bronchodilator FDA-approved to treat chronic obstructive pulmonary disease

(COPD). In asthma, it is used off-label as an alternative reliever medication in patients who cannot take a short-acting beta-2 agonist.[4] Tiotropium bromide, an inhaled long-acting anticholinergic bronchodilator, is also approved only for use in COPD. In patients with asthma uncontrolled on an ICS, addition of tiotropium has been as effective as adding the LABA salmeterol in improving lung function and symptoms.[14] In one study, addition of tiotropium to combination treatment with an ICS and a LABA improved lung function in patients with poorly controlled severe asthma.[15]

Adverse effects of anticholinergics include dry mouth, pharyngeal irritation, increased intraocular pressure and urinary retention. They should be used with caution in patients with glaucoma, prostatic hypertrophy or bladder neck obstruction.

THEOPHYLLINE

Theophylline, taken alone or concurrently with an ICS, is now used infrequently for persistent asthma. Monitoring serum theophylline concentrations is recommended to maintain peak levels between 10 and 15 mcg/mL.

Adverse effects of theophylline include nausea, vomiting, nervousness, headache and insomnia. At high serum concentrations, hypokalemia, hyperglycemia, tachycardia, cardiac arrhythmias, tremor, neuromuscular irritability, seizures and death can occur. Many other drugs used concomitantly can interact with theophylline, either by increasing its metabolism and decreasing its serum concentrations and efficacy, or by decreasing its metabolism, leading to higher concentrations and toxicity.

ANTI-IgE ANTIBODY (OMALIZUMAB)

Omalizumab (*Xolair*) is a recombinant humanized monoclonal antibody that prevents IgE from binding to mast cells and basophils, thereby preventing release of inflammatory mediators after allergen

Continued on page 64

DRUGS FOR ASTHMA

Drug	Some Available Formulations
INHALED BETA-2 AGONISTS, SHORT-ACTING	
Albuterol – generic	Solution for nebulization[1]
single-dose vials	0.63, 1.25, 2.5mg/3mL 100 mg/20 mL
multi-dose vials	
AccuNeb (Dey)	Solution for nebulization[1]
single-dose vials	0.63, 1.25 mg/3 mL
ProAir HFA (Teva)	HFA MDI (200 inh/unit)
Proventil HFA (Schering)	90 mcg/inhalation
Ventolin HFA (GSK)	
Levalbuterol – generic	Solution for nebulization[1]
Xopenex (Sepracor)	0.31, 0.63, 1.25 mg/3 mL
Xopenex HFA (Sepracor)	HFA MDI (80, 200 inh/unit) 45 mcg/inh
Pirbuterol[2] – *Maxair Autohaler*	Breath-actuated CFC MDI (80, 400 inh/unit)
(Medicis)	200 mcg/inh
INHALED CORTICOSTEROIDS	
Beclomethasone dipropionate –	
QVAR (Teva)	HFA MDI (100 inh/unit) 40, 80 mcg/inhalation
Budesonide – *Pulmicort Flexhaler*	DPI (60, 120 inh/unit) 90, 180 mcg/inhalation
(AstraZeneca)	
Pulmicort Turbuhaler	DPI (200 inh/unit) 200 mcg/inhalation
	Susp for nebulization[4]
generic – single-dose vials	0.25, 0.5 mg/2mL
Pulmicort Respules (AstraZeneca)	
single-dose ampules	0.25, 0.5mg, 1mg/2mL
Ciclesonide – *Alvesco*	HFA MDI (60 inh/unit)
(Nycomed)	80, 160 mcg/inhalation
Flunisolide – *Aerospan* HFA	HFA MDI (60, 120 inh/unit)
(Forest)	80 mcg/inhalation

CFC = Chlorofluorocarbon; DPI = Dry powder inhaler; HFA = Hydrofluoroalkane;
MDI = Metered-dose inhaler
1. Nebulized solutions may be more convenient for very young, very old and other patients unable to use pressurized aerosols. More time is required to administer the drug, however, and the device is usually not portable.

Adult Dosage	Pediatric Dosage
1.25-5 mg q4-8h PRN	2-4 yrs: 0.63-2.5 mg q4-6h PRN 5-11 yrs: 1.25-5 mg q4-8h PRN
	2-12 yrs: 0.63 or 1.25 mg tid-qid PRN
90-180 mcg q4-6h PRN	$\geq$4 yrs: 90-180 mcg q4-6h PRN
0.63-1.25 mg tid q6-8h PRN	6-11 yrs: 0.31-0.63 mg tid q6-8h PRN $\geq$12 yrs: 0.63-1.25 mg tid q6-8h PRN
90 mcg q4-6h PRN	$\geq$4 yrs: 90 mcg q4-6h PRN
200-400 mcg q4-6h PRN	$\geq$12 yrs: 200-400 mcg q4-6h PRN
40-320 mcg bid[3]	5-11 yrs: 40-80 mcg bid[3]
360-720 mcg bid	6-17 yrs: 180-360 mcg bid
200-800 mcg bid[3]	$\geq$6 yrs: 200-400 mcg bid[3]
————	1-8 yrs: 0.25-0.5 mg once/d or bid or 1 mg once/d[3]
80-320 mcg bid[3]	$\geq$12 yrs: 80-320 mcg bid[3]
160-320 mcg bid[3]	6-11 yrs: 80-160 mcg bid[3]

2. CFC-containing MDIs will not be marketed after December 2013.
3. Dose is based on prior asthma therapy. See package insert for specific dosing instructions.
4. Only approved for use in children 1-8 years old.

Continued on next page.

Drugs for Asthma

DRUGS FOR ASTHMA (continued)

Drug	Some Available Formulations
INHALED CORTICOSTEROIDS (continued)	
Fluticasone propionate –	
Flovent Diskus (GSK)	DPI (60 inh/unit) 50, 100, 250 mcg/blister
Flovent HFA (GSK)	HFA MDI (120 inh/unit) 44, 110, 220 mcg/inhalation
Mometasone furoate –	
Asmanex Twisthaler (Schering-Plough)	DPI (30, 60, 120 inh/unit) 110, 220 mcg/inhalation
ORAL GLUCOCORTICOIDS	
Methylprednisolone – generic	4, 8, 16, 32 mg tabs
Medrol (Pfizer)	
Prednisolone – generic	5, 15 mg/5 mL syrup
Prelone (Teva)	15 mg/5 mL syrup
Orapred (Shionogi)	15 mg/5 mL PO solution
Orapred ODT	10, 15, 30 mg disintegrating tabs
Pediapred (UCB)	5 mg/5mL PO solution
Prednisone – generic	1, 2.5, 5, 10, 20, 50 mg tabs; 5 mg/5 mL PO solution
INHALED BETA-2 AGONISTS, LONG-ACTING[5]	
Salmeterol – *Serevent Diskus* (GSK)	DPI (60 inh/unit) 50 mcg/blister
Formoterol – *Foradil Aerolizer* (Merck)	DPI (60 inh/unit) 12 mcg/capsule
INHALED CORTICOSTEROID/LONG-ACTING BETA-2 AGONIST COMBINATIONS	
Fluticasone/salmeterol –	
Advair Diskus (GSK)	DPI (60 inh/unit) 100, 250, 500 mcg/50 mcg per blister[6]
Advair HFA (GSK)	HFA MDI (60, 120 inh/unit) 45, 115, 230 mcg/21 mcg per inhalation
Budesonide/formoterol –	
Symbicort HFA (AstraZeneca)	HFA MDI (60, 120 inh/unit) 80, 160 mcg/4.5 mcg per inhalation

5. Use of a long-acting beta-2 agonist (LABA) alone without concomitant use of a long-term asthma controller medication is contraindicated in the treatment of asthma.

Adult Dosage	Pediatric Dosage
100-1000 mcg bid[3]	4-11 yrs: 50-100 mcg bid[3]
88-880 mcg bid[3]	4-11 yrs: 88 mcg bid
220-440 mcg 1x/day in evening or 220 mcg bid	4-11 yrs: 110 mcg 1x/d in evening
5-60 mg once/d or every other day **or** 40-60 mg once/d or divided bid x 3-10 days for an acute exacerbation	0-11 yrs: 0.25-2 mg/kg once/d or every other day (max 60 mg/d) **or** 1-2 mg/kg x 3-10 days (max 60 mg/d) for an acute exacerbation
50 mcg bid	$\geq$4 yrs: 50 mcg bid
12 mcg bid	$\geq$5 yrs: 12 mcg bid
1 inhalation bid	4-11 yrs: 1 inhalation (100/50 mcg) bid $\geq$12 yrs: 1 inhalation bid
2 inhalations bid	$\geq$12 yrs: 2 inhalations bid
2 inhalations bid	$\geq$12 yrs: 2 inhalations bid

6. Only the 100 mcg/50 mcg formulation is approved for use in children.

Continued on next page.

DRUGS FOR ASTHMA (continued)

Drug	Some Available Formulations
INHALED CORTICOSTEROID/LONG-ACTING BETA-2 AGONIST COMBINATIONS (continued)	
Mometasone/formoterol –	
Dulera (Merck)	HFA MDI (120 inh/unit)
	100, 200 mcg/5 mcg per inhalation
LEUKOTRIENE MODIFIERS[7]	
Montelukast – *Singulair* (Merck)	10 mg tabs, 4, 5 mg chew tabs,
	4 mg oral granules
Zafirlukast – generic	10, 20 mg tabs
Accolate (AstraZeneca)	
Zileuton – *Zyflo* (Cornerstone)	600 mg tabs
extended-release	
Zyflo CR	600 mg ER tabs
ANTICHOLINERGICS[9]	
Ipatropium – generic	Solution for nebulization[1] 250 mcg/mL
Atrovent HFA	HFA MDI (200 inh/unit) 17 mcg/inhalation
(Boehringer Ingelheim)	
Tiotropium – *Spiriva HandiHaler*	DPI (5, 30, 90 inh/unit) 18 mcg/capsule
(Boehringer Ingelheim)	
ANTI-IGE ANTIBODY	
Omalizumab – *Xolair* (Genentech)	Powder for injection 150 mg/5 mL vial
THEOPHYLLINE	
generic	100, 125, 200, 300 mg ER caps;
	100, 200, 300, 400, 450, 600 mg ER tabs;
	80 mg/15mL oral elixir[11]
Theo-24 (UCB Pharma)	100, 200, 300, 400 mg ER caps[11]
Uniphyl (Purdue)	400, 600mg ER tabs[11]

7. Montelukast is taken once daily in the evening, with or without food. Montelukast granules must be taken within 15 minutes of opening the packet. Zafirlukast is taken 1 hour before or 2 hours after a meal. Zileuton is taken within one hour after morning and evening meals.
8. Montelukast is approved for prevention of exercise-induced bronchoconstriction only in patients ≥15 years. Dosage for 12-23 months: one packet of 4-mg oral granules; for 2-5 yrs: 4-mg chewable tab once/d or one packet of 4 mg oral granules; for 6-14 yrs: 5-mg chewable tab once/d.
9. Not FDA-approved for asthma.

Adult Dosage	Pediatric Dosage
2 inhalations bid	$\geq$12 yrs: 2 inhalations bid
10 mg PO once/d	$\geq$1 yr: 4 or 5 mg PO once/day[8]
20 mg PO bid	5-11 yrs: 10 mg PO bid
	$\geq$12 yrs: 20 mg PO bid
600 mg PO qid	$\geq$12 yrs: 600 mg PO qid
1200 mg PO bid	$\geq$12 yrs: 1200 mg PO bid
500 mcg qid PRN	——
2 inhalations qid PRN	——
18 mcg once/d	——
150-300 mg SC q4wks or 225-375 mg SC q2wks[10]	$\geq$12 yrs: 150-300 mg q4wks or 225-375 mg q2wks[10]
300-600 mg/once day or divided bid	10 mg/kg/d[12]
300-600 mg once/day	
400-600 mg once/day	

10. Dose depends on the patient's body weight and total serum IgE level. See package insert for specific dosing instructions.
11. Extended-release formulations may not be interchangeable. If Theo-24 is taken <1 hr before a high fat meal, the entire 24-hour dose can be released in a 4-hour period.
12. Starting dose. Usual maximum is 16 mg/kg/day in children >1 year old; in infants 0.2 x (age in weeks) + 5 = dose in mg/kg/day.

exposure. It is FDA-approved for use in patients ≥ 12 years old with moderate to severe persistent asthma not well controlled on an ICS who have well-documented specific sensitization to a perennial airborne allergen, such as mold or animal dander.

Subcutaneous injection of omalizumab every 2 or 4 weeks reduces asthma exacerbations and has a modest ICS-sparing effect. In adults and adolescents, when added to standard treatment, omalizumab improved symptoms and reduced exacerbations.[16,17] When added to standard treatment in children with allergic asthma, omalizumab improved asthma control, decreased exacerbations and reduced maintenance ICS doses.[18] Use of omalizumab does not preclude simultaneous use of allergen immunotherapy.

Adverse Effects – Injection-site pain and bruising occur in up to 20% of patients. Anaphylaxis has occurred, but the incidence is extremely low (0.2% of patients). A national task force monitoring these rare cases of anaphylaxis continues to advise keeping patients under observation for 2 hours after the first three omalizumab injections, and for 30 minutes after subsequent injections. Additionally, patients receiving omalizumab should be instructed on how to recognize anaphylaxis and told to self-inject epinephrine promptly if it occurs.[19]

IMMUNOTHERAPY

In selected patients with allergic asthma, specific immunotherapy ("allergy shots") may provide long-lasting benefits in reducing asthma symptoms and the need for medications.[20]

BRONCHIAL THERMOPLASTY

Approved by the FDA in 2010 for use in adults with severe persistent asthma not well controlled on an ICS and a LABA, bronchial thermoplasty has been shown to modestly improve lung function and asthma symptoms.[21] Patients undergo fiber optic bronchoscopy on 3 separate occasions 3 weeks apart. During the procedure, the walls of the central airways are treated with radiofrequency energy that is converted to heat (target tissue temperature 65°C), resulting in ablation of airway smooth muscle. Adverse effects, mainly worsening of asthma, are common in the weeks immediately following bronchial thermoplasty. A long-term study found that lung function appears to remain stable for at least 5 years following the procedure.[22]

TREATMENT FAILURE

Failure of pharmacologic treatment can usually be attributed to lack of adherence to prescribed medications, uncontrolled co-morbid conditions or continued exposure to tobacco smoke and other airborne pollutants, allergens or irritants. Smoking and exposure to second-hand smoke can cause airway hyperresponsiveness and decrease the effectiveness of ICSs. Some patients with asthma may concurrently be taking aspirin or other NSAIDs that can cause asthma symptoms. Oral or topical nonselective beta-adrenergic blockers, such as propranolol (*Inderal*, and others) or timolol, can precipitate bronchospasm in patients with asthma and decrease the bronchodilating effect of beta-2 agonists.

Patients with moderate or severe asthma may benefit from meeting with trained asthma educators to have their inhaler technique checked and develop a personalized asthma management plan.[23]

MANAGING EXACERBATIONS

Intensifying treatment at home when symptoms begin can prevent exacerbations from becoming severe. Self-management of asthma exacerbations, guided by a written asthma action plan, generally calls for increased doses of a SABA and, sometimes, initiation of a short course of an oral glucocorticoid. Doubling the dose of an ICS is not effective and quadrupling the dose is only marginally effective.[24]

Treatment of acute asthma in the urgent care setting or emergency department generally involves supplemental oxygen to relieve hypoxemia and a SABA (sometimes in combination with ipratropium), usually administered by face mask and nebulizer. In moderate or severe exacerbations, an oral or intravenous glucocorticoid is added to reduce airway inflammation. Severe asthma exacerbations unresponsive to these measures may respond to intravenous magnesium sulphate, especially in children, or to inhalation of heliox (typically a mixture of helium 79% and oxygen 21%) to decrease airflow resistance and improve delivery of aerosolized medications.[25]

EXERCISE-INDUCED BRONCHOCONSTRICTION

Exercise-induced bronchoconstriction (EIB) may be the only manifestation of asthma in patients with mild disease. EIB may also be a transient phenomenon in non-asthmatic athletes.[26] SABAs used just before exercise will prevent EIB for 2-3 hours after inhalation in most patients. LABAs prevent EIB for up to 12 hours, but if they are taken regularly, the protection may wane and not last throughout the day. Montelukast decreases EIB in up to 50% of patients within 2 hours after administration; the protection may last for up to 24 hours and does not wane with repeated use. In some patients, EIB occurs because of poorly-controlled persistent asthma; in these patients, daily anti-inflammatory medications should be started or increased in dosage.[3]

ASTHMA IN PREGNANCY

Maternal asthma increases the risk of pregnancy-related complications including pre-eclampsia, perinatal mortality, preterm birth and low birth weight.[27] Albuterol is the preferred SABA for use in pregnancy. ICSs (budesonide is the best studied) are the preferred long-term controller medications in pregnancy; they do not appear to cross the placenta or have any effects on fetal adrenal function and are therefore unlikely to have adverse effects on fetal growth and development.[27,28] The safety of low-to-moderate doses of ICSs has been confirmed in a cohort study of 13,280 pregnancies; the incidence of major congenital malformations was increased with use of higher ICS doses (>1000 mcg/day beclomethasone equivalent) during the first trimester.[29] LABAs and montelukast appear to be safe in pregnancy.[30] Teratogenicity in animals has been reported with zileuton.

ASTHMA IN CHILDREN

For children with mild intermittent asthma, a SABA should be used as needed. For mild, moderate or severe persistent asthma, ICSs are the preferred long-term treatment for control of symptoms; ICSs do not, however, alter the underlying severity or progression of the disease. In young children, a SABA or an ICS may best be delivered through a metered-dose inhaler with a valved holding chamber and face mask or mouthpiece, or through a nebulizer. Dry powder inhalers are not suitable for use in young children, who cannot reliably inhale rapidly or deeply enough to use them effectively. Nebulized budesonide is FDA-approved for use in children as young as one year of age. ICSs given in low doses for years are generally safe for use in children, but linear growth should be monitored. Low- or medium-dose ICSs administered regularly may reduce growth velocity slightly during the first year of treatment, but final adult height does not appear to be affected.[7]

Montelukast can be used as the controller in children whose parents prefer not to use an ICS. It may also be used instead of a LABA as an add-on to an ICS, but it is generally less effective.

ASTHMA IN THE ELDERLY

Asthma in the elderly is often associated with co-morbidities, such as cardiovascular disease, diabetes, dementia, depression and frailty, and with polypharmacy. Elderly asthmatic patients are more likely to have fixed airway obstruction with features that overlap COPD. The elderly have more adverse effects from ICSs, including skin bruising, cataracts, increased intraocular pressure, hyperglycemia and accelerated loss of bone mass. They may have both a reduced response to beta-adrenergic bronchodilators, especially if concomitantly taking a beta blocker, and an increased incidence of tachycardia, arrhythmias and tremors. In these patients, tiotropium can be a useful bronchodilator. Some older patients have difficulty inhaling any medication from a metered-dose or dry-powder inhaler and may require a nebulizer.[31-33]

ASTHMA AND CO-MORBID DISEASES

Asthma is often associated with other co-morbid conditions including allergic rhinitis, gastroesophageal reflux disease (GERD), obesity, sinusitis, depression and anxiety. Such co-morbidities can make asthma more difficult to treat.[34]

Allergic Rhinitis – Up to 95% of patients with asthma also suffer from persistent rhinitis. Concurrent pharmacologic treatment of both asthma and rhinitis improves asthma outcomes.[35] Patients with concomitant allergic rhinitis and allergic asthma may benefit from specific immunotherapy with standardized allergens.[20]

GERD – Patients with poorly controlled asthma have a higher prevalence of GERD, but no cause-and-effect relationship has been demonstrated. In asthma patients who have concomitant GERD symptoms, treatment with a proton pump inhibitor may slightly improve pulmonary function and asthma-related quality of life.[36] In asthma patients with asymptomatic GERD, treatment with a proton pump inhibitor does not improve asthma control.[37]

Obesity – Obesity has been associated with asthma persistence and severity.[4] Overweight and obese asthmatic patients may have a diminished response to ICSs.[38] Weight loss may improve lung function and responsiveness to treatment. Bariatric surgery has been reported to improve asthma control and airway hyperresponsiveness in overweight adults.[39]

1. CH Fanta. Asthma. N Engl J Med 2009; 360:1002.
2. PM O'Byrne. Therapeutic strategies to reduce asthma exacerbations. J Allergy Clin Immunol 2011; 128:257.
3. JM Weiler et al. Pathogenesis, prevalence, diagnosis, and management of exercise-induced bronchoconstriction: a practice parameter. Ann Allergy Asthma Immunol 2010; 105 (6 suppl):S1.
4. National Heart, Lung and Blood Institute. National Asthma Education and Prevention Program (NAEPP). Expert Panel Report (EPR) 3. Guidelines for the diagnosis and management of asthma. Full Report 2007. Available at www.nhlbi.nih.gov/guidelines/asthma/index.htm. Accessed January 18, 2012.
5. RC Strunk et al. Long-term budesonide or nedocromil treatment, once discontinued, does not alter the course of mild to moderate asthma in children and adolescents. J Pediatr 2009; 154:682.
6. HW Kelly. Comparison of inhaled corticosteroids: an update. Ann Pharmacother 2009; 43:519.
7. S Pedersen. Clinical safety of inhaled corticosteroids for asthma in children: an update of long-term trials. Drug Saf 2006; 29:599.
8. PM O'Byrne et al. Risks of pneumonia in patients with asthma taking inhaled corticosteroids. Am J Respir Crit Care Med 2011; 183:589.
9. E Bateman et al. Meta-analysis: effects of adding salmeterol to inhaled corticosteroids on serious asthma-related events. Ann Intern Med 2008; 149:33.
10. RF Lemanske, Jr et al. Step-up therapy for children with uncontrolled asthma receiving inhaled corticosteroids. N Engl J Med 2010; 362:975.
11. AW McMahon et al. Age and risks of FDA-approved long-acting ß-adrenergic receptor agonists. Pediatrics 2011; 128:e1147.
12. BA Chowdhury et al. Assessing the safety of adding LABAs to inhaled corticosteroids for treating asthma. N Engl J Med 2011; 364:2473.
13. PM O'Byrne et al. Efficacy of leukotriene receptor antagonists and synthesis inhibitors in asthma. J Allergy Clin Immunol 2009; 124:397.
14. SP Peters et al. Tiotropium bromide step-up therapy for adults with uncontrolled asthma. N Engl J Med 2010; 363:1715.
15. HA Kerstjens et al. Tiotropium improves lung function in patients with severe uncontrolled asthma: a randomized controlled trial. J Allergy Clin Immunol 2011; 128:308.
16. GJ Rodrigo et al. Efficacy and safety of subcutaneous omalizumab vs placebo as add-on therapy to corticosteroids for children and adults with asthma: a systematic review. Chest 2011; 139:28.
17. NA Hanania et al. Omalizumab in severe allergic asthma inadequately controlled with standard therapy: a randomized trial. Ann Intern Med 2011; 154:573.

Drugs for Asthma

18. WW Busse et al. Randomized trial of omalizumab (anti-IgE) for asthma in inner-city children. N Engl J Med 2011; 364:1005.
19. L Cox et al. American Academy of Allergy, Asthma & Immunology/American College of Allergy, Asthma & Immunology Omalizumab-Associated Anaphylaxis Joint Task Force follow-up report. J Allergy Clin Immunol 2011; 128:210.
20. MA Calderón et al. Allergen-specific immunotherapy for respiratory allergies: from meta-analysis to registration and beyond. J Allergy Clin Immunol 2011; 127:30.
21. Bronchial thermoplasty for asthma. Med Lett Dugs Ther 2010; 52:65.
22. NC Thomson et al. Long-term (5 year) safety of bronchial thermoplasty: Asthma Intervention Research (AIR) trial. BMC Pulm Med 2011; 11:8.
23. FM Ducharme et al. Written action plan in pediatric emergency room improves asthma prescribing, adherence, and control. Am J Respir Crit Care Med 2011; 183:195.
24. J Oborne et al. Quadrupling the dose of inhaled corticosteroid to prevent asthma exacerbations: a randomized, double-blind, placebo-controlled, parallel-group clinical trial. Am J Respir Crit Care Med 2009; 180:598.
25. SC Lazarus. Emergency treatment of asthma. N Engl J Med 2010; 363:755.
26. V Bougault et al. Airway hyperresponsiveness in elite swimmers: is it a transient phenomenon? J Allergy Clin Immunol 2011; 127:892.
27. M Schatz and MP Dombrowski. Asthma in pregnancy. N Engl J Med 2009; 360:1862.
28. NA Hodyl et al. Fetal glucocorticoid-regulated pathways are not affected by inhaled corticosteroid use for asthma during pregnancy. Am J Respir Crit Care Med 2011; 183:716.
29. L Blais et al. High doses of inhaled corticosteroids during the first trimester of pregnancy and congenital malformations. J Allergy Clin Immunol 2009; 124:1229.
30. LN Bakhireva et al. Safety of leukotriene receptor antagonists in pregnancy. J Allergy Clin Immunol 2007; 119:618.
31. PG Gibson et al. Asthma in older adults. Lancet 2010; 376:803.
32. CE Reed. Asthma in the elderly: diagnosis and management. J Allergy Clin Immunol 2010; 126:681.
33. NA Hanania et al. Asthma in the elderly: Current understanding and future research needs—a report of a National Institute on Aging (NIA) workshop. J Allergy Clin Immunol 2011; 128:S4.
34. M Cazzola et al. Asthma and comorbid medical illness. Eur Respir J 2011; 38:42.
35. J Bousquet et al. Allergic rhinitis and its impact on asthma (ARIA) 2008 update (in collaboration with the World Health Organization, GA(2)LEN and AllerGen). Allergy 2008; 63 Suppl 86:8.
36. TO Kiljander et al. Effect of esomeprazole 40 mg once or twice daily on asthma: a randomized, placebo-controlled study. Am J Respir Crit Care Med 2010; 181:1042.
37. American Lung Association Asthma Clinical Research Centers et al. Efficacy of esomeprazole for treatment of poorly controlled asthma. N Engl J Med 2009; 360:1487.
38. E Forno et al. Decreased response to inhaled steroids in overweight and obese asthmatic children. J Allergy Clin Immunol 2011; 127:741.
39. AE Dixon et al. Effects of obesity and bariatric surgery on airway hyperresponsiveness, asthma control, and inflammation. J Allergy Clin Immunol 2011; 128:508.

DRUGS FOR
Chronic Obstructive Pulmonary Disease

Original publication date – November 2010

The goals of drug therapy for chronic obstructive pulmonary disease (COPD) are to reduce symptoms such as dyspnea, improve exercise tolerance and quality of life, and decrease complications of the disease such as acute exacerbations. Other guidelines for treatment of this condition have been published or updated in recent years.[1,2]

SMOKING CESSATION — The primary strategy for preventing and minimizing the risk of COPD is to help patients stop smoking. Cigarette smoking causes 85% of all COPD cases. Smoking cessation offers health benefits at all stages of the disease and can slow the decline of lung function. Counseling and pharmacotherapy can help patients stop smoking. Effective medications include varenicline *(Chantix)*, nicotine replacement therapies and bupropion *(Zyban*, and others).[3] Varenicline offers a unique mechanism of action as a partial nicotinic receptor agonist, but the current labeling includes precautions regarding possible neuropsychiatric side effects.[4] Combinations of smoking cessation therapies may offer additional benefit.[5]

INHALATION DEVICES — Guidelines are available for choosing among aerosol delivery devices.[6] Inhaled drugs are available in the US mainly in pressurized metered-dose inhalers (MDIs), which require a propellant, and dry powder inhalers (DPIs), which do not. Spacers used

Drugs for Chronic Obstructive Pulmonary Disease

SOME DRUGS FOR SMOKING CESSATION

Medication	Formulations	Daily Adult Maintenance Dose
NICOTINIC-ACETYLCHOLINE RECEPTOR AGONISTS		
Nicotine transdermal* *NicoDerm CQ*	7, 14, 21 mg/24 hr	1 patch/d
Nicotine nasal spray *Nicotrol NS*	0.5 mg/spray; 1 dose = 2 sprays	1 dose 8-40x/d
Nicotine oral inhaler *Nicotrol*	10 mg cartridge	4-16 cartridges/d
Nicotine polacrilex gum* *Nicorette*	2, 4 mg/piece	8-24 pieces/d
Nicotine polacrilex lozenge* *Commit*	2, 4 mg/lozenge	8-20 lozenges/d
DOPAMINERGIC-NORADRENERGIC REUPTAKE INHIBITOR		
Bupropion SR – generic	50, 100, 150, 200 mg sustained-release tabs	150 mg 2x/d
Zyban	150-mg sustained-release tabs	
NICOTINIC RECEPTOR PARTIAL AGONIST		
Varenicline – *Chantix*	0.5, 1 mg tabs	1 mg 2x/d

* Available without a prescription over-the-counter (OTC).

with MDIs may improve drug delivery, decrease mouth deposition, and require less hand-breath coordination. Nebulizers may be easier to use for some patients, such as the elderly, but more time is required to administer the drug with a nebulizer, and the device, which is usually not portable, requires greater care in cleaning.[7]

SHORT-ACTING BRONCHODILATORS — For patients with intermittent symptoms, therapy with an inhaled short-acting bronchodilator is recommended for acute relief. Typically, these patients have mild airflow obstruction and symptoms are usually associated with exertion. Short-acting agents, which include inhaled **beta$_2$-agonists** such as albuterol and the **anticholinergic** ipratropium, can relieve symptoms and improve exercise tolerance. Short-acting beta$_2$-agonists have a more rapid onset (<5 minutes) than ipratropium (15 minutes). With chronic use, short-acting beta$_2$-agonists have a duration of action of less than 4 hours, while ipratropium may continue to act for 6 hours (MDI) or as long as 8 hours (nebulized). There is no convincing evidence that any one of the inhaled short-acting beta$_2$-agonists is more effective than any other.

Combination Therapy – Combining a beta$_2$-agonist with ipratropium has an additive effect. The combination of ipratropium/albuterol has been more effective than either drug alone and is available in a single inhaler.

Adverse Effects – Beta$_2$-agonists can cause tachycardia, skeletal muscle tremors and cramping, headache, palpitations, prolongation of the QT interval, insomnia, hypokalemia and increases in serum glucose. They require caution in patients with cardiovascular disease; unstable angina and myocardial infarction have been reported. Tolerance to these effects occurs with chronic therapy.

Ipratropium is a quaternary ammonium anticholinergic agent with limited systemic absorption. The most common adverse effect is dry mouth. Pharyngeal irritation, urinary retention and increases in intraocular pressure may occur. Anticholinergics should be used with caution in patients with glaucoma and in those with symptomatic prostatic hypertrophy or bladder neck obstruction.

LONG-ACTING BRONCHODILATORS — For patients with evidence of significant airflow obstruction and chronic symptoms, regular treatment with a long-acting bronchodilator is recommended. Choices include an inhaled long-acting beta$_2$-agonist or an anticholinergic agent.

Drugs for Chronic Obstructive Pulmonary Disease

SOME INHALED SHORT-ACTING BRONCHODILATORS

Drug	Formulation
SHORT-ACTING BETA$_2$-AGONISTS[1]	
Albuterol	90 mcg/inhalation
generic	
Albuterol sulfate	
generic	
single-dose vials	2.5 mg base/3 mL
multi-dose vials	2.5 mg base/0.5 mL
AccuNeb	
single-dose vials	0.63 or 1.25 mg base/3 mL
ProAir HFA	90 mcg base/inhalation
Proventil HFA	
Ventolin HFA	
Levalbuterol hydrochloride	
generic	0.31, 0.63, 1.25 mg/3mL
Xopenex	
Levalbuterol tartrate	
Xopenex HFA	45 mcg/inhalation
Pirbuterol	
Maxair Autohaler	200 mcg/inhalation
SHORT-ACTING ANTICHOLINERGIC	
Ipratropium	
generic	250 mcg/mL
Atrovent HFA	17 mcg/inhalation
SHORT-ACTING BETA$_2$-AGONIST/SHORT-ACTING ANTICHOLINERGIC COMBINATION	
Albuterol sulfate/ipratropium	
Combivent	90 mcg albuterol base/18 mcg ipratropium/inhalation
DuoNeb	2.5 mg albuterol base/0.5 mg ipratropium/3 mL

HFA = Hydrofluoroalkane, MDI = Metered-dose inhaler
1. Not FDA-approved for use in COPD.

Delivery Device	Inhalations/ Unit	Usual Adult Dosage
MDI	200	2 inhalations q4-6h PRN
Nebulizer	—	2.5 mg q6-8h PRN
Nebulizer	—	2.5 mg q6-8h PRN
MDI	200	2 inhalations q4-6h PRN
Nebulizer	—	0.63-1.25 mg tid q6-8h
MDI	200	2 inhalations q4-6h PRN
MDI	80, 400	2 inhalations q4-6h PRN
Nebulizer	—	500 mcg qid PRN
MDI	200	2 inhalations qid PRN
MDI	200	2 inhalations qid PRN
Nebulizer	—	2.5 mg/0.5 mg qid PRN (max 6 doses/d)

Drugs for Chronic Obstructive Pulmonary Disease

SOME INHALED LONG-ACTING BRONCHODILATORS

Drug	Formulation
LONG-ACTING BETA$_2$-AGONISTS	
Salmeterol – *Serevent Diskus*	50 mcg/blister
Formoterol – *Foradil Aerolizer*	12 mcg/capsule
Perforomist	20 mcg/2 mL
Arformoterol – *Brovana*	15 mcg/2 mL
LONG-ACTING ANTICHOLINERGIC	
Tiotropium – *Spiriva HandiHaler*	18 mcg/capsule
CORTICOSTEROID/LONG-ACTING BETA$_2$-AGONIST COMBINATIONS	
Fluticasone/salmeterol – *Advair Diskus*[1]	100, 250, 500 mcg/50 mcg/blister
Advair HFA[2]	45, 115, 230 mcg/21 mcg/inhalation
Budesonide/formoterol – *Symbicort*[3]	80, 160 mcg/4.5 mcg/inhalation
Mometasone/formoterol – *Dulera*[2]	100, 200 mcg/5 mcg/ inhalation

DPI = Dry powder inhaler, HFA = Hydrofluoroalkane, MDI = Metered-dose inhaler
1. Only the 250/50 mcg dose is FDA-approved for use in COPD.

Long-acting beta$_2$-agonists are intended to provide sustained bronchodilation for at least 12 hours. They have been shown to improve lung function and quality of life and to lower exacerbation rates in patients with COPD.[7]

All long-acting beta$_2$-agonist products in the US include a boxed warning about an increased risk of asthma-related deaths; there is no evidence to date that patients with COPD are at risk. The adverse effects of long-acting beta$_2$-agonists are similar to those of the short-acting agents. Tolerance to the therapeutic effects of long-acting beta$_2$-agonists can occur with continued use.

Tiotropium is the only long-acting anticholinergic agent available in the US. Its long duration of action allows once-daily dosing, and there is no

Delivery Device	Inhalations/ Unit	Usual Adult Dosage
DPI	60	50 mcg bid
DPI	60	12 mcg bid
Nebulizer	—	20 mcg bid
Nebulizer	—	15 mcg bid
DPI	30	18 mcg once/d
DPI	60	1 inhalation bid
MDI	120	2 inhalations bid
MDI	120	2 inhalations bid
MDI	120	2 inhalations bid

2. Only FDA-approved for treatment of asthma.
3. Only the 160/4.5 mcg dose is FDA-approved for use in COPD.

evidence of tolerance to its therapeutic benefits. The UPLIFT trial enrolled 5993 patients with COPD and randomized them to either tiotropium or placebo, in addition to their usual medications, for 4 years. Spirometry, quality-of-life scores, and exacerbation and hospitalization rates all improved compared to placebo in tiotropium-treated patients, but treatment did not reduce the rate of decline in forced expiratory volume in one second (FEV_1) during the study period.[8,9] Tiotropium is generally well tolerated and appears to be safe.[10] Adverse effects are similar to those of ipratropium.[11]

Combination Therapy – When patients are not adequately controlled with a single long-acting bronchodilator, combining tiotropium with a long-acting beta$_2$-agonist may be helpful.[12]

THEOPHYLLINE — Slow-release theophylline can be used as an oral alternative or in addition to inhaled bronchodilators (see Table). Its primary mechanism of action is bronchodilation. Because of significant inter- and intra-patient variability in theophylline clearance, dosing requirements vary. The drug has a narrow therapeutic index; monitoring is warranted periodically to maintain serum concentrations between 5 and 12 mcg/mL for treatment of COPD.

Adverse Effects – At theophylline serum concentrations higher than 12-15 mcg/mL, nausea, nervousness, headache and insomnia occur with increasing frequency in patients with COPD. Vomiting, hypokalemia, hyperglycemia, tachycardia, cardiac arrhythmias, tremors, neuromuscular irritability and seizures can also occur at higher serum concentrations. Theophylline is metabolized in the liver, primarily by CYP1A2 and CYP3A4. Any drug that is an inhibitor or inducer of these enzymes can affect theophylline metabolism.[13] Clearance of theophylline is reduced in the elderly and in patients with liver disease or heart failure.

CORTICOSTEROIDS — In patients with severe COPD (FEV_1 <50%) who experience frequent exacerbations while receiving one or more long-acting bronchodilators, addition of an **inhaled** corticosteroid is recommended to reduce the number of exacerbations. In the 3-year, double-blind TORCH study of more than 6000 patients with COPD, the combination of salmeterol/fluticasone reduced exacerbation frequency by 25% compared to placebo, and by 12% compared to salmeterol alone.[14] The results of several large, international studies indicate that inhaled corticosteroids do not slow the progression of COPD.[15]

Adverse Effects – Risks of **inhaled** corticosteroid therapy are dose-related. Local effects on the mouth and pharynx include candidiasis and dysphonia. Systemic absorption of inhaled corticosteroids has been associated with skin bruising, cataracts, reduced bone mineral density and an increased risk of fractures. Several large studies have found an

THEOPHYLLINE

Drug	Formulations	Usual Adult Dosage
THEOPHYLLINE		
generic	450 mg ER tabs; 100, 125, 200, 300 mg ER caps[1]	300-600 mg/day
Theo-24	100, 200, 300, 400 mg ER caps[1]	
Theochron	100, 200, 300, 450 mg ER tabs[1]	

ER = extended-release
1. Extended-release formulations may not be interchangeable. If *Theo-24* is taken with food, the entire 24-hour dose is released in a 4-hour period.

increased risk of pneumonia associated with high doses (1000 mcg/day) of fluticasone.[16]

Long-term treatment with **oral** corticosteroids is not recommended in COPD. The risks of such treatment include myopathy, glucose intolerance, weight gain and immunosuppression.

TRIPLE-THERAPY REGIMENS — Two short-term studies (2-12 weeks) have demonstrated a benefit with triple therapy (tiotropium, formoterol or salmeterol, and fluticasone or budesonide) compared to 1 or 2 agents in relieving symptoms such as dyspnea and in improving lung function.[17,18] In one of these studies, the number of severe exacerbations decreased by 62% with triple therapy. In a retrospective cohort study, the triple-combination regimen reduced overall mortality by 40%.[19]

OXYGEN THERAPY — For patients with severe hypoxemia, use of long-term supplemental oxygen therapy has been shown to increase survival and quality of life.[20] Oxygen therapy may also increase exercise capacity in patients with mild or moderate hypoxemia, but its long-term benefits in such patients are unclear.[21]

SOME INHALED CORTICOSTEROIDS

Drug	Formulation
CORTICOSTEROIDS[1]	
Beclomethasone dipropionate	
QVAR HFA	40, 80 mcg/inhalation
Budesonide – generic	0.25, 0.5 mg/2 mL
Pulmicort Respules	0.25, 0.5, 1 mg/2 mL
Pulmicort Flexhaler	90, 180 mcg/inhalation
Pulmicort Turbuhaler	200 mcg/inhalation
Flunisolide	
Aerospan HFA[2]	80 mcg/inhalation
Fluticasone propionate	
Flovent Diskus	50, 100, 250 mcg/blister
Flovent HFA	44, 110, 220 mcg/inhalation
Mometasone furoate	
Asmanex Twisthaler	110, 220 mcg/inhalation
Triamcinolone acetonide	
Azmacort	75 mcg/inhalation
CORTICOSTEROID/LONG-ACTING BETA$_2$-AGONIST COMBINATIONS	
Fluticasone/salmeterol	
Advair Diskus[3]	100, 250, 500 mcg/50 mcg/blister
Advair HFA[1]	45, 115, 230 mcg/21 mcg/inhalation
Budesonide/formoterol[4]	
Symbicort	80, 160 mcg/4.5 mcg/inhalation
Mometasone/formoterol –	100, 200 mcg/5 mcg/inhalation
Dulera[1]	

N.A. Not available
DPI = Dry powder inhaler, HFA = Hydrofluoroalkane (propellant), MDI = Metered-dose inhaler
1. Only FDA-approved for treatment of asthma.

Delivery Device	Inhalations/ Unit	Usual Adult Dosage
MDI	100	40-320 mcg bid
Nebulizer	—	250-500 mcg 1x/d or bid or 1.0 mg 1x/d
DPI	60, 120	360-720 mcg bid
DPI	200	200-800 mcg bid
MDI	60, 120	160-320 mcg bid
DPI	60	100-500 mcg bid
MDI	120	88-440 mcg bid
DPI	30, 60, 120	220-440 mcg 1x/d or bid (max 880 mcg/d)
MDI	240	150 mcg tid-qid or 300 mcg bid
DPI	60	1 inhalation bid
MDI	120	2 inhalations bid
MDI	120	2 inhalations bid
MDI	120	2 inhalations bid

2. FDA-approved for maintenance treatment of asthma.
3. Only the 250/50 mcg dose is FDA-approved for use in COPD.
4. Only the 160/4.5 mcg dose is FDA-approved for use in COPD.

IMMUNIZATIONS — Patients with COPD should receive influenza vaccine and pneumococcal vaccine to reduce their risk of infection and complications from these pathogens.[22]

PULMONARY REHABILITATION — The benefits of pulmonary rehabilitation programs are well established for patients with COPD. Pulmonary rehabilitation can reduce dyspnea and improve functional capacity and quality of life, as well as reduce the number of hospitalizations.[23]

ACUTE EXACERBATIONS — A major focus of the chronic treatment of COPD is to reduce the frequency and severity of exacerbations, which have a significant effect on the course of the disease. When exacerbations occur, treatment includes intensification of short-acting bronchodilators, short-term therapy with systemic corticosteroids, and usually a course of antimicrobial therapy. Short-acting $beta_2$-agonists are generally used first. Among patients requiring hospitalization, oral prednisone doses of 40-60 mg daily for up to two weeks appeared to be as effective as more aggressive corticosteroid dosing.[24] The use of ventilatory support and supplemental oxygen therapy has been shown to reduce the morbidity and mortality associated with acute exacerbations.[20]

SUMMARY — Patients with COPD should stop smoking; pharmacotherapy may be helpful, especially with varenicline *(Chantix)*. Patients with mild, intermittent symptoms can be treated with inhaled short-acting bronchodilators for symptom relief. When symptoms become more severe or persistent, inhaled long-acting bronchodilators may be used. Regular use of long-acting bronchodilators can decrease the number of acute exacerbations. Combinations of a $beta_2$-agonist with an anticholinergic can be used for patients inadequately controlled with a single agent. For patients with severe COPD who experience frequent exacerbations, addition of an inhaled corticosteroid (triple therapy) is recommended. For patients with severe hypoxemia, oxygen therapy can improve survival.

Drugs for Chronic Obstructive Pulmonary Disease

1. KF Rabe et al. Global strategy for the diagnosis, management, and prevention of chronic obstructive pulmonary disease: GOLD Executive Summary. Updated 2009. Available at www.goldcopd.com. Accessed September 22, 2010.
2. BR Celli et al. Standards for the diagnosis and treatment of patients with COPD: a summary of the ATS/ERS position paper. Eur Respir J 2004; 23:932. Updated 2005. Available at www.thoracic.org. Accessed August 18, 2010.
3. Drugs for tobacco dependence. Treat Guidel Med Lett 2008; 6:61.
4. RS McIntyre. Varenicline and suicidality: a new era in medication safety surveillance. Expert Opin Drug Saf 2008; 7:511.
5. R Strassmann et al. Smoking cessation interventions in COPD: a network meta-analysis of randomized trials. Eur Respir J 2009; 34:634.
6. MB Dolovich et al. Device selection and outcomes of aerosol therapy: Evidence-based guidelines: American College of Chest Physicians/American College of Asthma, Allergy, and Immunology. Chest 2005; 127:335.
7. GJ Rodrigo et al. Safety of long-acting beta-agonists in stable COPD. A systematic review. Chest 2008; 133:1079.
8. DP Tashkin et al. A 4-year trial of tiotropium in chronic obstructive pulmonary disease. N Engl J Med 2008; 359:1543.
9. M Decramer et. al. Effect of tiotropium on outcomes in patients with moderate chronic obstructive pulmonary disease (UPLIFT): a prespecified subgroup analysis of a randomized controlled trial. Lancet 2009; 374:1171.
10. TM Michele. The safety of tiotropium – the FDA's conclusions. N Engl J Med 2010; 363:1097.
11. Tiotropium (Spiriva) for COPD. Med Lett Drugs Ther 2004; 46:41.
12. DP Tashkin et al. Formoterol and tiotropium compared with tiotropium alone for treatment of COPD. COPD 2009; 6:17.
13. DA Flockhart. Drug interactions: cytochrome P450 drug interaction table. Indiana School of Medicine (2007). Available at http://medicine.iupui.edu/clinpharm/ddis/table.asp. Accessed September 22, 2010.
14. PM Calverley et al. Salmeterol and fluticasone propionate and survival in chronic obstructive pulmonary disease. N Eng J Med 2007; 356:775.
15. IA Yang et al. Inhaled corticosteroids for stable chronic obstructive pulmonary disease. Cochrane Database Syst Rev 2007; (2):CD002991.
16. Safety of inhaled corticosteroids in chronic obstructive pulmonary disease (COPD). Med Lett Drugs Ther 2010; 52:41.
17. T Welte et al. Efficacy and tolerability of budesonide/formoterol added to tiotropium in patients with chronic obstructive pulmonary disease. Am J Respir Crit Care Med 2009; 180:741.
18. D Singh et al. Superiority of triple therapy with salmeterol/fluticasone proprionate and tiotropium bromide versus individual components in moderate to severe COPD. Thorax 2008; 63:592.

19. TA Lee. Outcomes associated with tiotropium use in patients with chronic obstructive pulmonary disease. Arch Intern Med 2009; 169:1403.
20. GF Joos. Are beta$_2$-agonists safe in patients with acute exacerbations of COPD? Am J Respir Crit Care Med 2007; 176:322.
21. MB Drummond and RA Wise. Oxygen therapy in COPD: what do we know? Am J Respir Crit Care Med 2007; 176:321.
22. Adult immunization. Treat Guidel Med Lett 2009; 51:27.
23. R Casaburi et al. Pulmonary rehabilitation for management of chronic obstructive pulmonary disease. N Engl J Med 2009; 360:1329.
24. PK Lindenauer et al. Association of corticosteroid dose and route of administration with risk of treatment failure in acute exacerbation of chronic obstructive pulmonary disease. JAMA 2010; 303:2359.

ROFLUMILAST *(DALIRESP)* FOR COPD

Originally published in The Medical Letter – July 2011; 53:59

Roflumilast (*Daliresp* – Forest), an oral phosphodiesterase 4 (PDE4) in-hibitor, was approved by the FDA to reduce the risk of exacerbations in adult patients with severe chronic obstructive pulmonary disease (COPD) associated with chronic bronchitis and a history of exacerbations.

STANDARD TREATMENT — The goals of drug therapy for COPD are to reduce symptoms such as dyspnea, improve exercise tolerance and quality of life, and decrease complications of the disease such as acute exacerbations. COPD exacerbations may hasten progression of the disease and lead to early mortality.

Patients with mild, intermittent COPD symptoms can be treated with an inhaled short-acting bronchodilator for symptom relief. When symptoms become more severe or persistent, an inhaled long-acting bronchodilator may be used. Combinations of a beta$_2$-agonist with an anticholinergic can be used for patients inadequately controlled with a single agent. For patients with severe COPD who experience frequent exacerbations, addition of an inhaled corticosteroid (triple therapy) is recommended.[1]

MECHANISM OF ACTION — Roflumilast is a selective inhibitor of PDE4, an enzyme involved in the metabolism of cyclic adenosine monophosphate (cAMP) in inflammatory cells. Inhibition of PDE4 leads to increased intracellular levels of cAMP and a reduction in inflammation. Roflumilast is not a bronchodilator.

PHARMACOKINETICS — Roflumilast is 80% bioavailable. It is extensively metabolized; both the parent drug and an N-oxide metabolite are responsible for the therapeutic effects. The area under the concentration-time curve for the active metabolite is 10 times greater than that of the parent drug, but the metabolite is 3 times less potent as a PDE4 inhibitor.

Drugs for Chronic Obstructive Pulmonary Disease

The terminal half-life is 17 hours for roflumilast and 30 hours for the N-oxide metabolite.

CLINICAL STUDIES — In 2 double-blind, placebo-controlled trials, a total of 3091 patients with severe or very severe COPD associated with chronic bronchitis and at least one COPD exacerbation requiring systemic glucocorticosteroids or hospitalization within the past year were randomized to roflumilast 500 mcg once daily or placebo for 52 weeks.[2] Use of long-acting anticholinergic drugs or corticosteroids was not allowed during the trial. Prebronchodilator FEV_1 increased by 48 mL compared to placebo, and the annual rate per patient of moderate to severe exacerbations was significantly lower in patients treated with roflumilast (1.14 vs. 1.37). Roflumilast also significantly improved postbronchodilator FEV_1 compared to placebo, but did not lower overall mortality.

In studies in patients with less severe disease, roflumilast did not significantly reduce exacerbations compared to placebo.[3,4] Roflumilast has not been compared with other drugs for this indication.

ADVERSE EFFECTS — In clinical trials, diarrhea and nausea have been the most common adverse effects leading to discontinuation of roflumilast. Weight loss has been reported in 7.5% of patients treated with the drug compared to 2.1% of placebo-treated patients. In the studies described above, patients in the roflumilast group lost a mean of 2.09 kg compared to a gain of 0.08 kg in the placebo group.[2] After discontinuation of the drug, patients often regained some of the lost weight. Psychiatric effects such as insomnia, depression and anxiety occurred in about 6% of patients taking roflumilast in clinical trials; suicidal ideation and completed suicide have been reported. Roflumilast is classified as category C (risk cannot be ruled out) for use during pregnancy.

DRUG INTERACTIONS — Roflumilast is metabolized by CYP3A4 and 1A2; drugs that are inhibitors of CYP3A4 or inhibit both CYP3A4 and 1A2, such as cimetidine, erythromycin, ketoconazole and fluvoxamine, can increase concentrations of roflumilast. Strong inducers of cytochrome P450 enzymes, such as rifampin and carbamazepine, can reduce the efficacy of roflumilast and should be avoided.

DOSAGE AND COST — The recommended dosage of roflumilast is 500 mcg once daily. No dose adjustment is recommended for patients with renal impairment, but moderate to severe hepatic impairment is a contraindication to its use. A month's supply (30 tablets) of roflumilast costs $207.00.[5]

CONCLUSION — Roflumilast *(Daliresp)*, the first oral phosphodiesterase-4 (PDE4) inhibitor, modestly improved lung function and reduced the number of moderate to severe exacerbations in patients with severe COPD associated with bronchitis. Nausea and diarrhea are common adverse effects, and psychiatric symptoms and weight loss can occur. Roflumilast should probably be reserved for patients not responding to other therapies.

1. Drugs for chronic obstructive pulmonary disease. Treat Guidel Med Lett 2010; 8:83.
2. PM Calverley et al. Roflumilast in symptomatic chronic obstructive pulmonary disease: two randomized clinical trials. Lancet 2009; 374:685.
3. PM Calverley et al. Effect of 1-year treatment with roflumilast in severe chronic obstructive pulmonary disease. Am J Respir Crit Care Med 2007; 176:154.
4. SI Rennard et al. Reduction of exacerbations by the PDE4 inhibitor roflumilast – the importance of defining different subsets of patients with COPD. Respir Res 2011; 12:18.
5. AWP listings according to *Price Alert* (July 15, 2011).

DRUGS FOR
Depression and Bipolar Disorder

Original publication date – May 2010 (revised March 2012)

Drugs are not the only treatment for mood disorders. Psychotherapy remains an important component in the management of these disorders, and electroconvulsive therapy (ECT) has a long history of efficacy and safety when drugs are ineffective, poorly tolerated or cannot be used. Some drugs are recommended here for indications that have not been approved by the FDA.

DRUGS FOR DEPRESSION

Antidepressant drugs produce a response in about 50-60% of adults with major depression and a remission in about 30%; 80% of patients will eventually respond to drug therapy. Antidepressants may take 1-4 weeks to produce detectable improvement and often require 6-12 weeks to achieve substantial benefit. Depression with psychotic features requires addition of an antipsychotic drug to an antidepressant or treatment with ECT.

SSRIs – Selective serotonin reuptake inhibitors (SSRIs), with their generally tolerable adverse effects and relative safety, are often used for treatment of major depression in both adults and children. There is no good evidence that any one SSRI is more effective than any other.[1] Fluoxetine is the only SSRI approved by the FDA for treatment of major

Drugs for Depression and Bipolar Disorder

SOME DRUGS FOR DEPRESSION

Drug	Formulations
SSRIs	
Citalopram – generic	10, 20, 40 mg tabs, caps; 40 mg ODT; 10 mg/5mL PO soln
Celexa (Forest)	10, 20, 40 mg tabs; 10 mg/5 mL PO soln
Escitalopram – *Lexapro* (Forest)	5, 10, 20 mg tabs; 5 mg/5 mL PO soln
Fluoxetine – generic	10, 20, 40 mg caps; 10, 20 mg tabs; 20 mg/5 mL PO soln
Prozac (Lilly/Dista)	10, 20, 40 mg caps
Prozac Weekly	90 mg cap
Paroxetine hydrochloride – generic	10, 20, 30, 40 mg tabs; 10 mg/5 mL
Paxil (GSK)	PO susp
extended release – generic	12.5, 25 mg tabs
Paxil CR	12.5, 25, 37.5 mg tabs
Paroxetine mesylate – *Pexeva* (Synthon)	10, 20, 30, 40 mg tabs
Sertraline – generic	25, 50, 100, 150, 200 mg tabs; 20 mg/mL PO concentrate
Zoloft (Pfizer)	25, 50, 100 mg tabs; 20 mg/mL PO concentrate
SNRIs	
Desvenlafaxine – *Pristiq* (Pfizer)	50, 100 mg tabs
Duloxetine – *Cymbalta* (Lilly)	20, 30, 60 mg caps
Venlafaxine – generic	25, 37.5, 50, 75, 100 mg tabs
Effexor (Pfizer)	
extended release – generic	37.5, 75, 150, 225 mg tabs
Effexor XR	37.5, 75, 150 mg caps
TCAs	
Amitriptyline – generic	10, 25, 50, 75, 100, 150 mg tabs
Desipramine – generic	10, 25, 50, 75, 100, 150 mg tabs
Norpramin (Sanofi-aventis)	
Imipramine – generic	10, 25, 50 mg tabs
Tofranil (Tyco)	
Tofranil PM	75, 100, 125, 150 mg caps
Nortriptyline – generic	10, 25, 50, 75 mg caps; 10 mg/5 mL
Pamelor (Tyco)	PO soln

Initial Daily Dosage	Usual Daily Dosage
20 mg once	40 mg once
10 mg once	10 mg once
10-20 mg once	20 mg once
90 mg 1x/wk	90 mg 1x/wk
20 mg once	20 mg once
12.5-25 mg once	25 mg once
10 mg once	20 mg once
50-100 mg once	50-200 mg once
50 mg once	50 mg once
20-30 mg bid	60 mg once or divided bid
25 mg tid	75 mg tid
37.5 mg once	225 mg once
50-100 mg once	150 mg once or divided
50-100 mg once	150 mg once or divided
25-50 mg once	100 mg once or divided
75-100 mg once	150 mg once or divided

Continued on next page.

SOME DRUGS FOR DEPRESSION (continued)

Drug	Formulations
MAOIs	
Isocarboxazid – *Marplan* (Validus)	10 mg tabs
Phenelzine – *Nardil* (Pfizer)	15 mg tabs
Selegiline – *Emsam* (BMS)	6, 9, 12 mg/24 hr patches
Tranylcypromine – generic	10 mg tabs
Parnate (GSK)	
OTHER	
Bupropion – generic	75, 100 mg tabs
Wellbutrin (GSK)	
extended release – generic	100, 150, 200, 300 mg tabs
Aplenzin (Sanofi-aventis)	174, 348, 522 mg tabs
Wellbutrin SR	100, 150, 200 mg tabs
Wellbutrin XL	150, 300 mg tabs
Mirtazapine – generic	7.5, 15, 30, 45 mg tabs
Remeron (Organon)	15, 30, 45 mg tabs
orally disintegrating – generic	15, 30, 45 mg tabs
Remeron SolTab	
Nefazodone – generic	50, 100, 150, 200, 250 mg tabs
Trazodone – generic	50, 100, 150, 300 mg tabs
extended release	
Oleptro (Labopharm)	150, 300 mg tabs

depressive disorder in children and adolescents; escitalopram is approved for treatment of depression in adolescents.

SNRIs — Venlafaxine is a serotonin and norepinephrine reuptake inhibitor (SNRI) for treatment of major depression; for most patients, SSRIs appear to be just as effective.[1] **Desvenlafaxine** is an active metabolite of venlafaxine with no demonstrated clinical advantage over the parent compound. **Duloxetine**, an SNRI also approved for treatment of diabetic neuropathy and fibromyalgia, is marketed particularly for treatment of

Initial Daily Dosage	Usual Daily Dosage
10 mg bid	30-40 mg divided
15 mg tid	30 mg bid
6 mg/24 hr	6, 9, 12 mg/24 hr
10 mg once	20-30 mg bid
100 mg bid	100 mg tid
150 mg once	150 mg bid
174 mg once	348 mg once
150 mg once	150 mg bid
150 mg once	300 mg once
15 mg hs	30-45 mg once
100 mg bid	200 mg bid
150 mg divided	300 mg divided
150 mg once	150-375 mg once

major depression in patients with prominent pain complaints, but its superiority over SSRIs for this indication is not well established.[2]

OTHER DRUGS — Tricyclic antidepressants (TCAs) and monoamine oxidase inhibitors (MAOIs) remain valuable alternatives for patients with moderate to severe depression who do not respond to or cannot tolerate an SSRI or SNRI. Selegiline, an MAOI used orally (*Eldepryl*, and others) to treat Parkinson's disease, has been approved by the FDA in a skin-patch formulation *(Emsam)* for treatment of major depression.[3]

Drugs for Depression and Bipolar Disorder

SSRI DRUG INTERACTION HIGHLIGHTS

Drug	CYP450[1,2]	Comments
Citalopram	Metabolized by 3A4, 2C19	Low potential for interactions
Escitalopram	Metabolized by 3A4, 2C19	Low potential for interactions
Fluoxetine	Metabolized by 2D6, 2C19 Potent inhibitor of 2D6 Moderate inhibitor of 2C19	Many interactions[2] Long half-life is a problem when interactions occur
Paroxetine	Metabolized by 2D6 Potent inhibitor of 2D6	Many interactions[2]
Sertraline	Metabolized by 2C19 Moderate inhibitor of 2D6	Low potential for interactions

1. See Med Lett Drugs Ther 2003; 45:46 for substrates, inducers and inhibitors of CYP450 isozymes.
2. See *The Medical Letter Adverse Drug Interactions Program.*

Bupropion is a useful alternative for depressed patients without severe anxiety who cannot tolerate the sexual dysfunction, weight gain and sedation that may occur with other antidepressants. **Mirtazapine**, which often is sedating, may be useful when insomnia or agitation is prominent, and its appetite-stimulating properties may be helpful in depressed patients with marked anorexia. **Nefazodone** is less frequently prescribed because of concerns about rare hepatotoxicity. **Trazodone**, which is also sedating, is commonly used as an adjunct to an SSRI in patients with insomnia.

ADVERSE EFFECTS — SSRIs – Jitteriness and insomnia early in treatment with SSRIs can be minimized by starting with low doses, possibly even lower than those recommended by the manufacturer for initial treatment. Other adverse effects associated with SSRIs include nausea, diarrhea, headache, dizziness, fatigue and sexual dysfunction (including decreased libido, impaired arousal and anorgasmia). Addition of sildenafil *(Viagra)* or bupropion has been helpful in treating some patients with SSRI-induced sexual dysfunction.[4] Some patients gain significant amounts of weight with continued SSRI use. When SSRIs are discontinued abruptly, withdrawal effects including nervousness, anxiety, irritability, electric-shock sensations, bouts of crying or tearfulness, dizziness, light-headedness, insomnia, confusion, trouble concentrating, nausea and vomiting can occur[5]; these effects are least likely to occur with fluoxetine. Use of SSRIs has caused hyponatremia in elderly patients and an increased risk of bleeding due to inhibition of serotonin uptake by platelets. Although generally considered safe in overdose, serotonin syndrome can develop. SSRIs have a variety of effects on CYP450 isoenzymes and may interact with many other drugs.[6] Citalopram, escitalopram and sertraline are least likely to interact.

SNRIs — The adverse effects of the SNRIs venlafaxine, desvenlafaxine and duloxetine are similar to those of SSRIs, but can also include increased sweating, tachycardia and (at least with duloxetine) urinary retention. Severe withdrawal symptoms can occur. SNRIs can cause a dose-dependent increase in blood pressure; blood pressure should be under control before starting the drug and monitored during treatment. Though uncommon, serious hepatotoxicity has been reported with duloxetine.[7]

Serotonin Syndrome – All SSRIs and SNRIs can, most commonly as a result of interactions with MAOIs, cause serotonin syndrome, a rare but potentially life-threatening condition characterized by altered mental status, fever, tachycardia, hypertension, agitation, tremor, myoclonus, hyperreflexia, ataxia, incoordination, diaphoresis, shivering and gastrointestinal symptoms. Some drugs with MAOI activity, such as the antimicrobial agent linezolid *(Zyvox)*, and some other serotonergic drugs, such as dextromethorphan, sumatriptan *(Imitrex)*, tramadol *(Ultram*, and others) and St. John's wort, may not be recognized as such, and can cause serotonin syndrome when taken concurrently with an SSRI or SNRI.[8]

Safety in Children – Adverse effects of SSRIs and SNRIs in children have been similar to those in adults, except that an increase in motor activity is more common in children. The long-term safety of these drugs, especially their effects on growth, personality development and behavior, is unknown. Concerns that SSRIs and SNRIs could cause depressed children or adolescents to consider or attempt suicide have led the FDA to require "black-box" warnings on all antidepressant drug labels, based on an FDA analysis of placebo-controlled antidepressant studies which found a greater risk of suicidal thoughts or behaviors (but not actually suicide) in children and young adults, though not in patients >24 years old. Expert clinicians believe that these drugs are much more likely to prevent suicide than to cause it. All depressed children, adolescents and adults, whether they are treated with drugs or not, should be monitored for suicidal ideation or behavior.

Other Drugs – TCAs commonly cause anticholinergic effects (urinary retention, constipation, dry mouth, blurred vision and confusion), orthostatic hypotension, weight gain, sedation and sexual dysfunction. They also can cause cardiac arrhythmias and may be lethal in overdose. Adverse effects of oral **MAOIs** include sleep disturbance, orthostatic hypotension, sexual dysfunction and weight gain, as well as potentially fatal interactions with SSRIs, sympathomimetics, and tyramine-rich foods resulting in hypertensive crisis or delirium.[6] The selegiline patch, when used at the lowest recommended dose (6 mg/24 hrs), appears to have no clinically meaningful interaction with tyramine-containing foods and does not cause sexual dysfunction, weight gain or hypotension. Drug-drug interactions can occur, however, with the patch and at higher doses, tyramine dietary modifications may be required.[3]

Bupropion can cause agitation, anxiety, insomnia, headache, nausea, anorexia and hypersensitivity reactions. Dose-related seizures may occur, especially in patients with eating disorders or other risk factors for seizure. **Mirtazapine** can cause sedation, increased appetite, weight gain, dizziness, dry mouth and constipation; febrile neutropenia has occurred rarely. **Nefazodone** has caused somnolence, dry mouth, nausea, dizziness, and rare, but life-threatening hepatic failure requiring liver transplantation, which has led to its withdrawal from the market in Canada and Europe. **Trazodone** can cause drowsiness, orthostatic hypotension and, rarely, priapism.

Mania – All antidepressants can induce mania in patients with bipolar disorder.

PREGNANCY — Maternal depression has itself been associated with delayed fetal development and low birth weight. Some studies have associated both SSRI exposure and untreated depression with an increase in preterm birth.[9,10] Infants born to mothers taking *SSRIs* in the third trimester have been reported to have a self-limited neonatal behavioral syndrome and a higher risk of requiring treatment in an intensive care unit, possibly related to withdrawal reactions, and of developing persistent pulmonary hypertension.[11] Some studies have shown an association of SSRIs with low birth weight and neonatal complications.[12] A retrospective study found an increased risk of major and cardiovascular malformations in infants born to mothers taking paroxetine, which has been reclassified by the FDA as category D (positive evidence of risk) for use in pregnancy.[13] Other studies have not shown an increased risk of cardiovascular malformations with paroxetine.[14] Small increases in septal heart defects have been reported with other SSRIs in pregnancy[15,16]; they are classified as category C (risk cannot be ruled out). Overall, risks of congenital malformations appear to be very low.[17,18]

Studies with **SNRIs** are limited,[15] but exposure during the third trimester may cause a self-limited neonatal behavioral syndrome.[19] **TCA** use in late pregnancy has been associated with jitteriness and convulsions in newborns. **MAOIs** have been associated with a few cases of teratogenicity. Data on other classes of antidepressants are lacking. Data on long-term behavioral effects of *in utero* antidepressant exposure are limited; one retrospective study found delays in sitting and walking (but within the normal range) in children exposed to antidepressants during pregnancy.[20]

CHOICE OF DRUGS — An SSRI is the initial treatment of choice for most patients with major depression, although an SNRI, bupropion (which has no sexual side effects), or mirtazapine could also be an appropriate first-line treatment. Since convincing comparative data on efficacy and adverse effects are lacking, the choice among SSRIs often is determined by their adverse effect profiles and differences in drug interactions. Generic citalopram or sertraline would be a reasonable first choice for treatment of depression in adults. Generic fluoxetine would be a good choice for drug treatment of depressed children or adolescents.

SECONDARY TREATMENT — When patients show only a partial response to an adequate trial of an SSRI after 2-4 weeks, many clinicians switch to another antidepressant, combine two antidepressants of different classes such as an SSRI and bupropion, or add another drug such as an atypical antipsychotic for "augmentation". MAOIs should not be added to an SSRI or SNRI because of the risk of serotonin syndrome.[8]

In one controlled trial, among patients with major depressive disorder who had not responded to or could not tolerate 12 weeks' treatment with the SSRI citalopram, **switching** to sustained-release bupropion, sertraline or extended-release venlafaxine led to remissions in 26%, 27% and 28% of patients respectively, but the study did not include a placebo group or one that continued on citalopram.[21]

Antipsychotic drugs may be useful for augmenting antidepressant agents when response is inadequate.[22] **Aripiprazole** and **quetiapine** have been approved by the FDA for adjunctive antidepressant treatment. A combination of **olanzapine** with fluoxetine has also been approved by the FDA for treatment-resistant depression and appears to be more effective than either drug alone.[23]

NONDRUG THERAPY — Psychotherapies, particularly cognitive behavioral therapy (CBT) and interpersonal therapy (IPT), are effective treatments for depression, but drug treatment is also indicated when depression is severe. ECT is effective for severe depression, depression with psychosis or bipolar disorder, and depression refractory to drugs; it can be used in pregnancy. The device division of the FDA has approved use of vagus nerve stimulation (VNS) for treatment-resistant depression, but its effectiveness is not clear.[24] Transcranial magnetic resonance stimulation is another non-pharmacological treatment that has been approved by the FDA for use in patients who have not responded to an antidepressant.[25] Unlike ECT, transcranial magnetic resonance stimulation does not require anesthesia and does not appear to have cognitive side effects, but its effectiveness is not well established and its availability is limited.[26]

MAINTENANCE THERAPY — The goal of antidepressant treatment is complete remission of symptoms; partial response is associated with an increased risk of relapse. For a first episode of depression, many experts recommend that antidepressant treatment continue at the same dose for at least 6-9 months following remission to consolidate recovery. For patients with recurrent depressive episodes, long-term maintenance therapy can reduce the risk of further recurrences.[27]

DRUGS FOR BIPOLAR DISORDER

Lithium continues to be the standard treatment for bipolar disorder, but antiepileptic drugs such as **valproate** and **carbamazepine** are also widely used despite evidence suggesting they are less effective in preventing recurrence.[28] **Atypical (second-generation) antipsychotic** drugs have received FDA approval for treatment of acute mania or mixed episodes, and for maintenance treatment of bipolar disorder. Quetiapine and the combination of olanzapine with fluoxetine have also been approved for treatment of depression associated with bipolar disorder, and the anticonvulsant lamotrigine has received FDA approval for prevention of recurrent depression in bipolar disorder. Monotherapy with antidepressant drugs can precipitate mania in patients with bipolar disorder.[29]

Drugs for Depression and Bipolar Disorder

SOME DRUGS FOR BIPOLAR DISORDER

Drug	Formulations
Aripiprazole – *Abilify* (BMS/Otsuka)[1-3]	2, 5, 10, 15, 20, 30 mg tabs; 10, 15 mg ODT; 1 mg/mL PO soln[4,11]
Asenapine – *Saphris* (Schering-Plough)[1,2]	5, 10 mg sublingual tabs
Carbamazepine – generic	100, 200, 300, 400 mg tabs; 100, 200 mg chewable tabs; 100 mg/5 mL PO susp[5]
Tegretol (Novartis)[6]	200 mg tabs; 100 mg chewable tabs; 100 mg/5 mL PO susp[5]
extended release – generic	100, 200, 400 mg tabs
Equetro (Validus)[1,2]	100, 200, 300 mg caps
Carbatrol (Shire)[6]	100, 200, 300 mg caps
Tegretol XR (Novartis)[6]	100, 200, 400 mg tabs
Olanzapine/fluoxetine – *Symbyax* (Lilly)[7]	3/25, 6/25, 6/50, 12/25, 12/50 mg olanzapine/fluoxetine caps
Lamotrigine[3] – generic	2, 5, 25, 50, 100, 150, 200, 250 mg tabs; 2, 5, 25 mg chewable tabs[9]
Lamictal (GSK)	25, 100, 150, 200 mg tabs; 25, 50, 100, 200 mg ODT; 2, 5, 25 mg chewable tabs[9]
Lithium[1,3] – generic	150, 300, 600 mg caps; 300 mg tabs; 8 mEq/5 mL PO soln
extended release – generic	300, 450 mg tabs
Lithobid SR (JDS)	300 mg tab
Olanzapine[1-3] – *Zyprexa* (Lilly)	2.5, 5, 7.5, 10, 15, 20 mg tabs[10]
orally disintegrating – *Zyprexa Zydis*	5, 10, 15, 20 mg tabs
Quetiapine – *Seroquel* (AstraZeneca)[1]	25, 50, 100, 200, 300, 400 mg tabs
extended release – *Seroquel XR*	50, 150, 200, 300, 400 mg tabs

1. FDA-approved for mania.
2. FDA-approved for mixed episode.
3. FDA-approved for maintenance treatment of bipolar disorder.
4. Aripiprazole PO solution should be given at the same dose (mg per mg) as the tablets, except that when patients receive the 30-mg tablet, 25 mg of the solution should be used.
5. Patients on conventional tablets can be switched to the suspension on a mg-per-mg basis, but in smaller, more frequent doses.
6. Not FDA-approved for bipolar disorder.

Initial Daily Dosage	Usual Daily Dosage
15 mg once	15-30 mg once
10 mg bid	10 mg bid
200-600 mg divided tid-qid	600-1200 mg divided bid or tid
200-600 mg divided tid-qid	600-1200 mg divided bid
6/25 mg once	6/25-12/50 mg once
25 mg once[8]	200 mg once
900-1800 mg divided tid	900-1200 mg divided tid or qid
900-1800 mg divided tid	900-1200 mg divided bid or tid
10 mg once	10-20 mg once
100-200 mg divided bid	400-800 mg divided bid
50-300 mg once	400-800 mg once

7. FDA-approved for depressive episode.
8. For monotherapy, titrate to a goal of 200 mg/day as follows: 25 mg/day for 2 weeks, then 50 mg/day for 2 weeks, then 100 mg/day for 1 week, then 200 mg/day.
9. Chewable tablets should be administered whole. If necessary, dose should be rounded down to the nearest whole tablet.
10. Also available in a form suitable for rapid intramuscular injection.
11. Also available as a long-acting injectable formulation.

Continued on next page.

Drugs for Depression and Bipolar Disorder

SOME DRUGS FOR BIPOLAR DISORDER (continued)

Drug	Formulations
Risperidone – generic	0.25, 0.5, 1, 2, 3, 4 mg tabs;
Risperdal (Janssen)[1,2]	1 mg/mL PO soln[11]
orally disintegrating – generic	0.25, 0.5, 1, 2, 3, 4 mg tabs
Risperdal M-Tab	0.5, 1, 2, 3, 4 mg tabs
Valproate[12]	
Valproic acid – generic	250 mg cap; 250 mg/5 mL
Depakene[6] (Abbott)	PO syrup
delayed release – *Stavzor* (Noven)	125, 250, 500 mg caps
Divalproex sodium – generic	125, 250, 500 mg tabs
Depakote[1] (Abbott)	
Depakote Sprinkle[6]	125 mg cap
extended release – *Depakote ER*[1]	250, 500 mg tabs
Ziprasidone – *Geodon* (Pfizer)[1,2,10]	20, 40, 60, 80 mg caps

12. Also available in an IV formulation as valproate sodium (*Depacon*, and others).
13. When switching from *Depakote* to *Depakote ER*, the dosage may need to be increased 8-20% to maintain serum concentrations.

EFFECTIVENESS — Antidepressants should be tapered and discontinued during a manic episode. For treatment of **acute mania**, lithium, valproate and atypical antipsychotics have similar efficacy.[27] Both lithium and valproate may take days to weeks to have a full therapeutic effect; acutely manic patients often require an antipsychotic drug or additional temporary treatment with a benzodiazepine.

For treatment of **depression in patients with bipolar disorder**, many studies have shown that lithium has protective effects against suicide and self-harm.[30] Other established treatments include the antipsychotic quetiapine[31] and the fixed-dose combination of olanzapine and fluoxetine. The effectiveness of valproate in treating depression in bipolar patients is unclear.[32] Patients who do not respond to first-line treatments for bipolar depression may benefit from lamotrigine.

102

Initial Daily Dosage	Usual Daily Dosage
2-3 mg once	4-6 mg once
250 mg tid	1500-2000 mg divided bid
750 mg divided	
750 mg divided	
25 mg/kg once[13]	25-40 mg/kg once[13]
40 mg bid	40-80 mg bid

Maintenance therapy with lithium alone or in combination with valproate, carbamazepine or lamotrigine decreases the risk of recurrent manic and depressive episodes. Lithium is more effective at preventing relapse than valproate alone.[33] A prospective randomized trial of lithium compared with valproate for maintenance therapy in rapid-cycling bipolar disorder found both to be equally effective in preventing relapse.[34] Second-generation antipsychotics are also effective in preventing recurrences of manic and depressive episodes, especially in combination with lithium. A long-acting form of risperidone, given intramuscularly every 2 weeks, has been approved by the FDA for maintenance treatment and may be helpful for patients with frequent relapse or in whom adherence is an issue.[35]

ADVERSE EFFECTS — Nausea and fatigue may occur in the first days to weeks of treatment with **lithium**, even when serum concentrations are

SOME ADVERSE EFFECTS OF SECOND-GENERATION ANTIPSYCHOTICS

Drug	Diabetes	Extrapyramidal Symptoms
Aripiprazole	+/–	+
Asenapine	++	+++
Clozapine*	++++	+/–
Olanzapine	++++	+
Quetiapine	+++	+/–
Risperidone	++	+++
Ziprasidone	+/–	+

*Clozapine is also associated with myocarditis and agranulocytosis; the other second-generation antipsychotics are not.

in the recommended range. Tremor, thirst, polyuria, edema and weight gain may persist for the duration of treatment. Lithium-induced tremors can be treated by lowering the dosage or adding a beta-blocker such as propranolol. Confusion and ataxia can occur when lithium levels are too high. Toxic renal effects, including tubular lesions, interstitial fibrosis and decreased creatinine clearance, have been reported with long-term use of lithium, but are uncommon. Nephrogenic diabetes insipidus, however, is common, increases the risk of further lithium toxicity, and may be irreversible.[36] Hypothyroidism is also common with long-term lithium treatment and can cause acute exacerbations of bipolar illness. Lithium may cause mild leukocytosis, can induce or exacerbate psoriasis, and can cause severe acne, folliculitis, hair loss and other skin reactions. Many commonly used drugs, including NSAIDs, ACE inhibitors and diuretics, can increase serum lithium concentrations; others, including theophylline and caffeine, can lower them.[37]

Adverse effects of **valproate** include sedation, weight gain, nausea, diarrhea and tremor, but tremor is less common than with lithium. Reversible

Elevated Prolactin	QTc Prolongation	Weight Gain
+/–	+/–	+
++	+	+
+/–	+	++++
+	+	++++
+/–	++	+++/++++
+++	+	+++
+	++	+/–

hair loss can occur. Thrombocytopenia has occurred and appears to be dose-related. Transient elevations of hepatic transaminases are common; fatal hepatotoxicity has occurred rarely, particularly in young children and with use of multiple anticonvulsants. Polycystic ovary syndrome has been reported in association with use of valproate.[38] Rare idiosyncratic reactions include hemorrhagic pancreatitis and agranulocytosis.

Adverse effects of **carbamazepine** include rash, dizziness, diplopia, nausea, somnolence, headache, hyponatremia and, rarely, Stevens-Johnson syndrome, agranulocytosis and aplastic anemia.[28] Carbamazepine has many adverse drug interactions. It is a strong inducer of CYP3A4 and can decrease serum concentrations and the effectiveness of drugs metabolized by this enzyme. It is also a CYP3A4 substrate, and serum concentrations can be increased to toxic levels by strong CYP3A4 inhibitors such as clarithromycin (*Biaxin*, and others).[6]

Adverse effects of **lamotrigine** include nausea, dizziness and somnolence. About 10% of patients develop mild rash; severe, life-threatening rash, including Stevens-Johnson syndrome and toxic epidermal necrolysis, has occured rarely.[39]

In addition to olanzapine and aripiprazole, **second-generation antipsychotics** used to treat bipolar disorder include asenapine, quetiapine, risperidone and ziprasidone. Somnolence is a common side effect. The FDA has required manufacturers of all second-generation antipsychotics to add a warning about an increased risk of death among elderly patients with dementia.

MONITORING — Use of **lithium** requires monitoring to maintain serum concentrations within the therapeutic range and avoid toxicity. Concentrations should be measured about 12 hours after the last dose. For acute treatment, target serum concentrations are 0.8 to 1.0 mEq/L. For maintenance, serum concentrations should be between 0.6 and 1.2 mEq/L. Renal function and thyroid function should be monitored routinely in patients taking lithium.

Liver function should be monitored in patients taking **valproate** and complete blood counts in patients taking **carbamazepine**. Serum concentrations of these drugs may be raised or lowered by other drugs taken concurrently.[6]

PREGNANCY — Discontinuation, especially abruptly, of mood stabilizer treatment is associated with an increased risk of mood episodes during pregnancy.[40] **Lithium** use during pregnancy has been associated with congenital cardiac abnormalities. High neonatal lithium concentrations are a risk factor for lower Apgar scores, longer hospital stays, and reversible neurologic toxicity that could be minimized or avoided by withholding maternal lithium for 24 hours before delivery. **Valproate** taken during pregnancy can cause neural tube defects, cardiac and other major teratogenic effects, adverse effects on neurocognitive development and neonatal toxicity; unless there is no alternative, it should not be used.[41-43] **Carbamazepine** is not recommended for use during pregnancy unless no alternatives exist, due to increased risk of major malformations including neural tube defects, low birth weight, and fetal and neonatal vitamin K deficiency, which can lead to neonatal hemorrhage. Data on use of **lamotrigine** in pregnancy are inconsistent; it appears to have a lower risk of adverse fetal outcomes than valproate or carbamazepine, but midline clefts have been reported.[44] Data on use of **second-generation antipsychotics** in pregnancy are limited, but increased birth weight (large for gestational age) has been reported.[45]

ALTERNATIVES — A **benzodiazepine** such as lorazepam (*Ativan*, and others) may be helpful when an adjunct is needed to sedate an agitated patient. Some clinicians have used **clozapine** to treat mania resistant to other drugs. **ECT** is effective for treatment of both acute mania and acute depression and may be particularly useful for drug-resistant mania and pregnant patients.

CHOICE OF DRUGS — Lithium, valproate, or a second-generation antipsychotic, alone or in combination with each other, are the drugs of choice for acute manic episodes and for maintenance treatment of bipolar disorder. Carbamazepine is an alternative. Lithium or quetiapine is preferred for treatment of depression in bipolar disorder. Lamotrigine in combination with lithium is an alternative for maintenance therapy of bipolar disorder, and it is a reasonable alternative to lithium alone or quetiapine for depressive episodes. Long-acting intramuscular risperidone can delay mood disorder relapse in patients with frequent episodes.[35]

1. G Gartlehner et al. Comparative benefits and harms of second-generation antidepressants: background paper for the American College of Physicians. Ann Intern Med 2008;149:734.
2. G Gartlehner et al. The general and comparative efficacy and safety of duloxetine in major depressive disorder: a systematic review and meta-analysis. Drug Saf 2009; 32:1159.
3. Transdermal selegiline (Emsam). Med Lett Drugs Ther 2006; 48:41.
4. R Balon. SSRI-associated sexual dysfunction. Am J Psychiatry 2006;163:1504.
5. EC van Geffen et al. Discontinuation symptoms in users of selective serotonin reuptake inhibitors in clinical practice: tapering versus abrupt discontinuation. Eur J Clin Pharmacol 2005; 61:303.
6. *The Medical Letter Adverse Drug Interactions Program.*

Drugs for Depression and Bipolar Disorder

7. J Wernicke et al. Hepatic effects of duloxetine-l: non-clinical and clinical trial data. Curr Drug Saf 2008; 3:132.
8. EW Boyer and M Shannon. The serotonin syndrome. N Engl J Med 2005; 352:1112.
9. KL Wisner et al. Major depression and antidepressant treatment: impact on pregnancy and neonatal outcomes. Am J Psychiatry 2009; 166:557.
10. N Lund et al. Selective serotonin reuptake inhibitor exposure in utero and pregnancy outcomes. Arch Pediatr Adolesc Med 2009; 163:949.
11. CD Chambers et al. Selective serotonin-reuptake inhibitors and risk of persistent pulmonary hypertension of the newborn. N Engl J Med 2006; 354:579.
12. H Nordeng and O Spigset. Treatment with selective serotonin reuptake inhibitors in the third trimester of pregnancy: effects on the infant. Drug Saf 2005; 28:565.
13. JA Cole et al. Bupropion in pregnancy and the prevalence of congenital malformations. Pharmacoepidemiol Drug Saf 2007; 16:474.
14. A Einarson et al. Evaluation of the risk of congenital cardiovascular defects associated with use of paroxetine during pregnancy. Am J Psychiatry 2008; 165:749.
15. A Einarson et al. Incidence of major malformations in infants following antidepressant exposure in pregnancy: results of a large prospective cohort study. Can J Psychiatry 2009; 54:242.
16. LH Pedersen et al. Selective serotonin reuptake inhibitors in pregnancy and congenital malformations: population based cohort study. BMJ 2009; 339:b3569.
17. S Alwan et al. Use of selective serotonin-reuptake inhibitors in pregnancy and the risk of birth defects. N Engl J Med 2007; 356:2684.
18. C Louik et al. First-trimester use of selective serotonin-reuptake inhibitors and the risk of birth defects. N Engl J Med 2007; 356:2675.
19. EL Moses-Kolko et al. Neonatal signs after late in utero exposure to serotonin reuptake inhibitors: literature review and implications for clinical applications. JAMA 2005; 293:2372.
20. LH Pedersen et al. Fetal exposure to antidepressants and normal milestone development at 6 and 19 months of age. Pediatrics 2010; 125:e600 Epub Feb 22.
21. AJ Rush et al. Bupropion-SR, sertraline, or venlafaxine-XR after failure of SSRIs for depression. N Engl J Med 2006; 354:1231.
22. JC Nelson and GI Papakostas. Atypical antipsychotic augmentation in major depressive disorder: a meta-analysis of placebo-controlled randomized trials. Am J Psychiatry 2009; 166:980.
23. MH Trivedi et al. An integrated analysis of olanzapine/fluoxetine combination in clinical trials of treatment-resistant depression. J Clin Psychiatry 2009; 70:387.
24. C Daban et al. Safety and efficacy of Vagus Nerve Stimulation in treatment-resistant depression. A systematic review. J Affect Disord 2008; 110:1.
25. DJ Schutter. Antidepressant efficacy of high-frequency transcranial magnetic stimulation over the left dorsolateral prefrontal cortex in double-blind sham-controlled designs: a meta-analysis. Psychol Med 2009; 39:65.
26. Repetitive transcranial magnetic stimulation (TMS) for medication-resistant depression. Med Lett Drugs Ther 2009; 51:11.

27. ME Thase and T Denko. Pharmacotherapy of mood disorders. Annu Rev Clin Psychol 2008; 4:53.
28. Extended-release carbamazepine (Equetro) for bipolar disorder. Med Lett Drugs Ther 2005; 47:27.
29. V Salvi et al. The use of antidepressants in bipolar disorder. J Clin Psychiatry 2008; 69:1307.
30. L Tondo and RJ Baldessarini. Long-term lithium treatment in the prevention of suicidal behavior in bipolar disorder patients. Epidemiol Psychiatr Soc 2009; 18:179.
31. ME Thase et al. Efficacy of quetiapine monotherapy in bipolar I and II depression: a double-blind, placebo-controlled study (the BOLDER II study). J Clin Psychopharmacol 2006; 26:600.
32. LA Smith et al. Valproate for the treatment of acute bipolar depression: systematic review and meta-analysis. J Affect Disord 2010; 122:1.
33. JR Geddes et al. Lithium plus valproate combination therapy versus monotherapy for relapse prevention in bipolar I disorder (BALANCE): a randomised open-label trial. Lancet 2010; 375:385.
34. JR Calabrese et al. A 20-month, double-blind, maintenance trial of lithium versus divalproex in rapid-cycling bipolar disorder. Am J Psychiatry 2005; 162:2152.
35. W Macfadden et al. A randomized, double-blind, placebo-controlled study of maintenance treatment with adjunctive risperidone long-acting therapy in patients with bipolar I disorder who relapse frequently. Bipolar Disorders 2009; 11:827.
36. JP Grunfeld and BC Rossier. Lithium nephrotoxicity revisited. Nat Rev Nephrol 2009; 5:270.
37. EM Grandjean and JM Aubry. Lithium: updated human knowledge using an evidence-based approach: part III: clinical safety. CNS Drugs 2009; 23:397.
38. L Bilo and R Meo. Polycystic ovary syndrome in women using valproate: a review. Gynecol Endocrinol 2008; 24:562.
39. H Arif et al. Comparison and predictors of rash associated with 15 antiepileptic drugs. Neurology 2007; 68:1701.
40. AC Viguera et al. Risk of recurrence in women with bipolar disorder during pregnancy: prospective study of mood stabilizer discontinuation. Am J Psychiatry 2007; 164:1817.
41. CL Harden et al. Practice parameter update: management issues for women with epilepsy—focus on pregnancy (an evidence-based review): teratogenesis and perinatal outcomes: report of the Quality Standards Subcommittee and Therapeutics and Technology Assessment Subcommittee of the American Academy of Neurology and American Epilepsy Society. Neurology 2009; 73:133.
42. KJ Meador et al. Cognitive function at 3 years of age after fetal exposure to antiepileptic drugs. N Engl J Med 2009; 360:1597.
43. T Tomson and D Battino. Teratogenic effects of antiepileptic medications. Neurol Clin 2009; 27:993.
44. DJ Newport et al. Lamotrigine in bipolar disorder: efficacy during pregnancy. Bipolar Disord 2008; 10:432.
45. JJ Newham et al. Birth weight of infants after maternal exposure to typical and atypical antipsychotics: prospective comparison study. Br J Psychiatry 2008; 192:333.

VILAZODONE *(VIIBRYD)* – A NEW ANTIDEPRESSANT

Originally published in The Medical Letter – July 2011; 53:53

Vilazodone (*Viibryd* – Forest), a selective serotonin reuptake inhibitor (SSRI) and partial $5\text{-}HT_{1A}$ receptor agonist, has been approved by the FDA for treatment of depression. It has been claimed to have no sexual side effects and not to cause weight gain.

RATIONALE — The manufacturer's premise is that addition of an agonist at $5\text{-}HT_{1A}$ could possibly lead to an earlier antidepressant effect and a decrease in SSRI-induced sexual side effects.[1] Buspirone (*Buspar*, and others), a $5\text{-}HT_{1A}$ agonist used for treatment of anxiety, has been tried as an add-on to an SSRI in patients not responding adequately to SSRI monotherapy.[2]

PHARMACOLOGY — Vilazodone peak serum concentrations are higher and the area under the concentration-time curve (AUC) is greater (64-85%) when the drug is taken with food. It is extensively metabolized in the liver, mainly by CYP3A4, and minimally excreted in urine and feces. The terminal half-life of vilazodone is about 25 hours.[3]

CLINICAL STUDIES — In a published trial in 410 adults with major depressive disorder, vilazodone 40 mg once daily was significantly more effective than placebo in reducing scores on the Montgomery-Asberg Depression Rating Scale (MADRS), the Hamilton Rating Scale for Depression (HAMD-17), and the Clinical Global Impressions of Severity of Illness (CGI-S) and Improvement (CGI-I) scales at 8 weeks. A significant difference from placebo was detectable after one week of treatment, which was the earliest time point of assessment.[4]

There are no published trials comparing vilazodone with any other antidepressant. SSRIs have also been reported to be effective after one week of use.[5]

ADVERSE EFFECTS — Diarrhea and nausea have been the most common short-term adverse effects of vilazodone. Insomnia, dizziness, headache, vomiting and dry eye have also occurred. Sexual side effects including decreased libido and abnormal orgasms have been reported. Vilazodone had no effect on body weight in the 8-week controlled trial; in a 52-week open-label trial, the mean change from baseline was +1.7 kgs.[6]

Vilazodone is classified as category C (risk cannot be ruled out) for use during pregnancy. Some infants born to mothers taking an SSRI during the 3rd trimester have been reported to have a neonatal behavioral syndrome and a higher risk of requiring treatment in an ICU and of developing persistent pulmonary hypertension.[7]

DRUG INTERACTIONS — Concurrent use of a strong CYP3A4 inhibitor, such as clarithromycin (*Biaxin*, and others), could increase plasma concentrations of vilazodone and its toxicity. Drugs that induce CYP3A4, such as rifampin, could reduce vilazodone plasma concentrations and decrease its effectiveness. Vilazodone, like other SSRIs, could increase the risk of GI bleeding, especially when taken with aspirin or another NSAID. Increased bleeding has been reported when SSRIs are co-administered with warfarin (*Coumadin*, and others). As with SSRIs, use of an MAO inhibitor is contraindicated within 14 days of taking vilazodone.

DOSAGE — The manufacturer recommends titrating the dose of vilazodone to improve its tolerability: 10 mg once daily during the first week, 20 mg during the second week, and 40 mg once daily, the recommended dose, beginning in the third week. Vilazodone should be taken with food to ensure adequate absorption. A maximum dose of 20 mg daily is recommended when vilazodone is taken concurrently with a strong inhibitor of CYP3A4. To avoid withdrawal symptoms and the risk of relapse, the dose of the drug should be reduced gradually when discontinuing therapy.[8]

SOME DRUGS FOR DEPRESSION

Drug	Some Formulations
SSRI AND 5-HT$_{1A}$	
Vilazodone – *Viibryd* (Forest)	10, 20, 40 mg tabs
SSRIs	
Citalopram – generic	10, 20, 40 mg tabs, caps; 10 mg/5mL PO soln
Celexa (Forest)	10, 20, 40 mg tabs; 10 mg/5 mL PO soln
Escitalopram – *Lexapro* (Forest)	5, 10, 20 mg tabs; 5 mg/5 mL PO soln
Fluoxetine – generic	10, 20, 40 mg caps; 10, 20 mg tabs; 20 mg/5 mL PO soln
Prozac (Lilly/Dista)	10, 20, 40 mg caps
weekly – generic	90 mg cap
Prozac Weekly	
Paroxetine hydrochloride – generic	10, 20, 30, 40 mg tabs; 10 mg/5 mL PO susp
Paxil (GSK)	
extended release – generic	12.5, 25, 37.5 mg tabs
Paxil CR	
Paroxetine mesylate –	10, 20, 30, 40 mg tabs
Pexeva (Synthon)	
Sertraline – generic	25, 50, 100 mg tabs; 20 mg/mL PO concentrate
Zoloft (Pfizer)	25, 50, 100 mg tabs; 20 mg/mL PO concentrate

1. Cost of 30 days' treatment with the lowest usual daily dose according to drugstore.com. Accessed July 5, 2011.
2. Generic prices can vary widely. A 30-day supply of generic citalopram, fluoxetine or paroxetine is available at some large retail pharmacies for $4.

CONCLUSION — The limited data available to date suggest that vilazodone *(Viibryd)* might be an effective antidepressant. There is no evidence that it acts more rapidly than SSRIs, causes fewer sexual side effects, or will not cause weight gain with long-term use. Until comparative data become available, an SSRI is preferred.

Initial Daily Dosage	Usual Daily Dosage	Cost[1]
10 mg once	40 mg once	$135.99
20 mg once	40 mg once	26.99[2]
		124.99
10 mg once	10 mg once	118.99
10-20 mg once	20 mg once	24.99[2]
		218.99
90 mg 1x/wk	90 mg 1x/wk	123.99
		153.99
20 mg once	20 mg once	15.99[2]
		121.99
12.5-25 mg once	25 mg once	105.86
		125.98
10 mg once	20 mg once	190.98
50-100 mg once	50-200 mg once	15.99[3]
		129.99

3. Cost of 30 100-mg tablets.

1. LA Dawson and JM Watson. Vilazodone: a 5-HT1A receptor agonist/serotonin transporter inhibitor for the treatment of affective disorders. CNS Neurosci Ther 2009; 15:107.
2. MH Trivedi et al. Medication augmentation after the failure of SSRIs for depression. N Engl J Med 2006; 354:1243.
3. A Khan. Vilazodone, a novel dual-acting serotonergic antidepressant for managing major depression. Expert Opin Investig Drugs 2009; 18:1753.

4. K Rickels et al. Evidence for efficacy and tolerability of vilazodone in the treatment of major depressive disorder: a randomized, double-blind, placebo-controlled trial. J Clin Psychiatry 2009; 70:326.
5. MJ Taylor et al. Early onset of selective serotonin reuptake inhibitor antidepressant action: systematic review and meta-analysis. Arch Gen Psychiatry 2006; 63:1217.
6. DS Robinson et al. A 1-year open-label study assessing the safety and tolerability of vilazodone in patients with major depressive disorder. Paper presented at the 163rd annual meeting of the American Psychiatric Association, New Orleans, LA, May 2010.
7. CD Chambers et al. Selective serotonin-reuptake inhibitors and risk of persistent pulmonary hypertension of the newborn. N Engl J Med 2006; 354:579.
8. RJ Baldessarini et al. Illness risk following rapid versus gradual discontinuation of antidepressants. Am J Psychiatry 2010; 167:934.

DRUGS FOR
Type 2 Diabetes

Original publication date – August 2011 (revised March 2012)

RECOMMENDATIONS: Used alone, oral hypoglycemic drugs generally lower glycated hemoglobin (A1C) by 0.5-1.5%. In the absence of contraindications, metformin is generally preferred as the first-line agent. If the desired goal is not achieved with metformin, addition of a sulfonylurea (glimepiride or glipizide) or pioglitazone could be considered. DPP-4 inhibitors are additional alternatives; long-term safety data are lacking, but their addition modestly reduces A1C and appears to be well tolerated. The GLP-1 agonists exenatide and liraglutide are injectable drugs that reduce A1C more than DPP-4 inhibitors. Most patients with type 2 diabetes eventually require multi-drug therapy or insulin. Some guidelines encourage early use of insulin if A1C remains poorly controlled on maximal-dose single-drug therapy.

The development of hyperglycemia in type 2 diabetes results from a combination of metabolic abnormalities that includes insulin resistance, diminished insulin secretion and excess hepatic glucose production. Diet, exercise and weight loss are helpful in improving glucose control, but most patients ultimately require drug therapy.[1]

BIGUANIDES — Metformin, (*Glucophage*, and others) the only biguanide marketed in the US, is generally prescribed first; it decreases hepatic glucose output and, to a lesser extent, increases peripheral glucose utilization. Metformin produces about the same reduction in A1C concentrations as a sulfonylurea (about 1-2%).

The United Kingdom Prospective Diabetes Study (UKPDS) found significant reductions in microvascular complications (retinopathy and nephropathy) in patients with type 2 diabetes treated intensively with a sulfonylurea, insulin or, in overweight patients, metformin, compared to patients treated with dietary restriction alone. After 10 years of post-study follow-up, the 342 patients treated with metformin during the study had 33% fewer myocardial infarctions and a 27% lower incidence of death than patients treated with dietary restriction, despite similar A1C levels soon after the study concluded.[2]

Adverse Effects – Metformin alone seldom causes hypoglycemia. Its favorable effect on body weight (typically weight neutral or weight loss of 2-3 kg) may be due partly to gastrointestinal adverse effects such as a metallic taste, nausea, diarrhea and abdominal pain, which can be minimized by starting with a low dose, increasing slowly, dividing doses and taking the drug with food. Long-term use of metformin can increase the risk of vitamin B12 deficiency.[3]

Lactic acidosis is a rare but potentially fatal complication. It can be avoided by not using metformin in patients with impaired renal function, other diseases that predispose to lactic acidosis (liver failure, major surgery, decompensated or acute heart failure) or alcoholism, or in those >80 years old if their renal function cannot be monitored. Metformin can be used in patients with stable heart failure.[4] It should be discontinued before radiographic studies with iodinated contrast, which can cause a temporary reduction in renal function, and should not be restarted until 48 hours later, after evaluating renal function. It is contraindicated in patients with renal impairment (serum creatinine ≥ 1.5 mg/dL in males, ≥ 1.4 mg/dL in females).

SULFONYLUREAS — The sulfonylureas **glimepiride** (*Amaryl*, and others), **glipizide** (*Glucotrol*, and others) and **glyburide** (*DiaBeta*, and others) interact with ATP-sensitive potassium channels in the beta-cell membrane to increase secretion of insulin. The commonly used second-generation agents are similar to each other in efficacy. A randomized, double-blind trial (the ADOPT study) in drug-naive patients with type 2 diabetes found that the incidence of monotherapy failure after 5 years was higher with glyburide (34%) than with metformin (21%) or rosiglitazone *(Avandia)* (15%).[5]

Adverse Effects – Sulfonylureas can cause weight gain and hypoglycemia, particularly in elderly patients with impaired renal or hepatic function. Glyburide appears to cause a higher incidence of hypoglycemia than glimepiride or glipizide.[6] In an analysis of 1310 patients with type 2 diabetes, use of a sulfonylurea before an MI was associated with lower post-MI mortality, compared to other therapies, but among the sulfonylurea-treated patients, use of glyburide was associated with a significantly higher mortality (7.5% vs. 2.7% with the other sulfonylureas).[7]

NON-SULFONYLUREA SECRETAGOGUES — **Repaglinide** *(Prandin)*[8] and **nateglinide** (*Starlix*, and others),[9] although structurally different from the sulfonylureas, also bind to ATP-sensitive potassium channels on beta cells and increase insulin release. Repaglinide is about as effective as the sulfonylureas in lowering A1C concentrations; nateglinide appears to be less effective.[10] Both repaglinide and nateglinide are rapidly absorbed and cleared, causing plasma levels of insulin to peak within 30 to 60 minutes. They must be taken before each meal; if a meal is missed, the dose should not be taken. Both are approved by the FDA for combined use with metformin or pioglitazone.

Adverse Effects – Hypoglycemia and weight gain occur with both repaglinide and nateglinide. Since both are at least partly metabolized by

Drugs for Type 2 Diabetes

CYP3A4, inhibitors of this enzyme, such as clarithromycin (*Biaxin*, and others), may increase their serum concentrations, and inducers, such as rifampin (*Rifadin*, and others), may decrease them. Both must be used with caution in patients with moderate to severe liver disease.

THIAZOLIDINEDIONES (TZDs) — Pioglitazone *(Actos)* and **rosiglitazone** decrease A1C concentrations by increasing the insulin sensitivity of adipose tissue, skeletal muscle and the liver. They can take 4 to 14 weeks to achieve their maximum effect. They are FDA-approved for use as monotherapy or in combination with metformin, a sulfonylurea or insulin (only pioglitazone). Whether the benefits of these agents outweigh their risks is unclear.

Cardiovascular Adverse Effects – The cardiovascular safety of thiazolidinediones is controversial.[11] A meta-analysis found an increased risk of myocardial infarction with rosiglitazone.[12] Both rosiglitazone and pioglitazone increase the risk of congestive heart failure[13]; their use is containdicated in class III or IV heart failure.

In two large retrospective cohort studies of elderly patients >65 years old with type 2 diabetes (total n = 267,307), rosiglitazone was associated with higher rates of stroke, heart failure and death compared to pioglitazone.[14,15] As a result, the FDA has severely restricted access to rosiglitazone; as of November 18, 2011, rosiglitazone-containing products will be available only to patients enrolled in the Avandia-Rosiglitazone Medicines Access Program.[16]

Other Adverse Effects – TZDs can cause peripheral edema; macular edema has also been reported. Weight gain is common; over a period of 6-12 months, mean weight gain has been 2-3 kg and can be much higher. Combination therapy with insulin can lead to even greater weight gain. TZDs have also been associated with reduced bone mineral density and an increased incidence of fractures, especially among women.[17] Since an earlier TZD was withdrawn from the market because of hepatic toxicity, the FDA recommends checking serum alanine aminotransferase (ALT) levels before starting TZD therapy and periodically thereafter; these drugs should not be used in patients with ALT levels >2.5 times the upper limit of normal. An increased risk of bladder cancer has been reported with high doses and long-term use of pioglitazone; it has been removed from the market in Germany and France.[18]

ALPHA-GLUCOSIDASE INHIBITORS — Acarbose (*Precose*, and others) and **miglitol** *(Glyset)* inhibit the alpha-glucosidase enzymes that line the brush border of the small intestine, interfering with hydrolysis of carbohydrates and delaying absorption of glucose and other monosaccharides. To lower postprandial glucose concentrations, these drugs must be taken with each meal.

Adverse Effects – Unabsorbed carbohydrates cause abdominal pain, diarrhea and flatulence due to osmotic effects and bacterial fermentation; slow titration can minimize these effects. Acarbose in high doses has been associated rarely with moderate transaminase elevations; miglitol has not. Fatal hepatic failure has been reported with acarbose. Given alone, neither of these drugs causes hypoglycemia, but use with either a sulfonylurea or insulin may increase the risk. Patients who develop hypoglycemia while taking these drugs should be treated with oral glucose because alpha-glucosidase inhibitors interfere with the breakdown of sucrose. Acarbose and miglitol are contraindicated in patients with chronic intestinal diseases, inflammatory bowel disease, colonic ulceration or any degree of intestinal obstruction.

INCRETIN-BASED AGENTS — Ingestion of a meal leads to release of the incretin hormones glucagon-like peptide 1 (GLP-1) and glucose-dependent insulinotropic polypeptide (GIP) from the gut. Both analogs of GLP-1 and inhibitors of dipeptidyl peptidase-4 (DPP-4), the enzyme that degrades GLP-1 and GIP, are now used to treat type 2 diabetes. These hormone-based agents potentiate insulin synthesis and release by pancreatic beta cells and decrease glucagon production by pancreatic alpha

Continued on page 124

SOME DRUGS FOR TYPE 2 DIABETES MELLITUS

Drug	Formulation
BIGUANIDE	
Metformin[2] – generic	500, 850, 1000 mg tabs
Glucophage (Bristol-Myers Squibb)	
extended-release – generic	500, 750 mg tabs
Glucophage XR (Bristol-Myers Squibb)	500, 750 mg tabs
Glumetza (Depomed)	500, 1000 mg tabs
Fortamet (Andryx)	500, 1000 mg tabs
liquid – *Riomet* (Ranbuxy)	500 mg/5 mL (4, 16 oz)
SECOND-GENERATION SULFONYLUREAS	
Glimepiride – generic	1, 2, 4, 8 mg tabs
Amaryl (Sanofi-Aventis)	1, 2, 4 mg tabs
Glipizide – generic	5, 10 mg tabs
Glucotrol (Pfizer)	
extended-release – generic	2.5, 5, 10 mg tabs
Glucotrol XL	
Glyburide – generic	1.25, 1.5, 2.5, 3, 5, 6 mg tabs
DiaBeta (Sanofi-Aventis)	1.25, 2.5, 5 mg tabs
Micronase (Pfizer)	1.25, 2.5, 5 mg tabs
micronized tablets – generic	1.5, 3, 4.5, 6 mg tabs
Glynase Prestab (Pfizer)	1.5, 3, 6 mg tabs
NON-SULFONYLUREA SECRETAGOGUES	
Nateglinide – generic	60, 120 mg tabs
Starlix (Novartis)	
Repaglinide – *Prandin* (Novo Nordisk)	0.5, 1, 2 mg tabs
THIAZOLIDINEDIONES	
Pioglitazone – *Actos* (Takeda)	15, 30, 45 mg tabs
Rosiglitazone – *Avandia* (GlaxoSmithKline)	2, 4, 8 mg tabs

1. FDA pregnancy categories: B = no evidence of risk in humans; C = risk cannot be ruled out.
2. Metformin is contraindicated in patients with renal impairment (serum creatinine ≥1.5 mg/dL in males, ≥1.4 mg/dL in females).
3. Should be taken with meals.
4. Once-daily dose should be given with the evening meal.

Pregnancy Category[1]	Usual Daily Dosage
B	1500-2550 mg PO divided[3]
	1500-2000 mg PO once[4]
	500-2000 mg PO once[4]
	1500-2500 mg PO once[4]
	1500-2550 mg PO divided[3]
C	1-4 mg PO once[5]
C	10-20 mg PO once or divided[6]
	5-20 mg PO once
B	5-20 mg PO once or divided[5]
C	
B	
B	1.5-12 mg PO once or divided[5]
C	60-120 mg PO tid[7]
C	1-4 mg PO tid[7,8]
C	15-45 mg PO once
C	4-8 mg PO once or divided

5. Once-daily dose should be given with breakfast or first meal.
6. Doses >15 mg/day should be divided bid.
7. Doses should be taken 15-30 minutes prior to meals.
8. A dose of 0.5 mg tid with meals is recommended for patients with severe renal impairment.

Continued on next page.

Drugs for Type 2 Diabetes

SOME DRUGS FOR TYPE 2 DIABETES MELLITUS (continued)

Drug	Formulation
ALPHA-GLUCOSIDASE INHIBITORS	
Acarbose – generic	25, 50, 100 mg tabs
Precose (Bayer)	
Miglitol – *Glyset* (Pfizer)	25, 50, 100 mg tabs
DPP-4 INHIBITORS	
Sitagliptin – *Januvia* (Merck)	25, 50, 100 mg tabs
Saxagliptin – *Onglyza* (Bristol-Myers Squibb)	2.5, 5 mg tabs
Linagliptin – *Tradjenta* (Boehringer Ingelheim)	5 mg tabs
GLP-1 AGONISTS	
Exenatide –	
immediate-release	
Byetta (Amylin/Lilly)	250 mcg/mL (1.2, 2.4 mL
extended-release	prefilled pen)
Bydureon (Amylin)	2 mg powder for injectable
	suspension
Liraglutide – *Victoza* (Novo Nordisk)	6 mg/mL (3 mL prefilled pen)
OTHER	
Colesevelam – *Welchol* (Sankyo)	625 mg tabs
Bromocriptine – *Cycloset* (VeroScience)	0.8 mg tabs
Pramlintide – *Symlin* (Amylin/Lilly)	1000 mcg/mL (1.5, 2.7 mL
	prefilled pen)
COMBINATION PRODUCTS	
Metformin/glipizide – generic	250/2.5, 500/2.5, 500/5 mg tabs
Metaglip (Bristol-Myers Squibb)	
Metformin/glyburide – generic	250/1.25, 500/2.5, 500/5 mg tabs
Glucovance (Bristol-Myers Squibb)	
Metformin/linagliptin – *Jentadueto*	500/2.5, 850/2.5, 1000/2.5 mg
(Boehringer Ingelheim)	tabs

9. Not recommended in patients with a serum creatinine >2 mg/dL.
10. A dose of 50 mg once daily is recommended for patients with a CrCl of $\geq$30-50 mL/min; 25 mg once daily is recommended for <30 mL/min.
11. A dose of 2.5 mg once daily is recommended for patients with a CrCl <50 mL/min.
12. Starting dose is 5 mcg twice daily, up to an hour before the morning and evening meals. After a month, the dose can be increased to 10 mcg twice daily.

Pregnancy Category[1]	Usual Daily Dosage
B	50-100 mg PO tid[3]
B	50-100 mg PO tid[3,9]
B	100 mg PO once[10]
B	2.5-5 mg PO once[11]
B	5 mg PO once
C	5 or 10 mcg SC bid before breakfast and dinner[12,13]
C	2 mg SC 1x/week[13]
C	1.2 or 1.8 mg SC once
B	3.8 g PO once or divided bid
B	1.6-4.8 mg PO once[3]
C	60-120 mcg SC tid immediately before main meals[14]
C	500 mg/2.5 mg PO bid[2,3]
B	500 mg/5 mg PO bid[2,3]
B	1 tab PO bid[2,3]

13. Not recommended in patients with a CrCl <30 mL/min; caution is recommended in renal transplant patients.
14. Dose for patients with type 2 diabetes.

Continued on next page.

SOME DRUGS FOR TYPE 2 DIABETES MELLITUS (continued)

Drug	Formulation
COMBINATION PRODUCTS (continued)	
Metformin/pioglitazone – generic	500/15, 850/15 mg tabs
Actoplus Met (Takeda)	
Actoplus Met XR	1000/15, 1000/30 mg tabs
Metformin/repaglinide – *Prandimet*	500/1, 500/2 mg tabs
(Novo Nordisk)	
Metformin/rosiglitazone – *Avandamet*	500/2, 500/4, 1000/2,
(GlaxoSmithKline)	1000/4 mg tabs
Glimepiride/rosiglitazone –	
Avandaryl (GlaxoSmithKline)	1/4, 2/4, 4/4, 2/8, 4/8 mg tabs
Glimepiride/pioglitazone – *Duetact* (Takeda)	2/30, 4/30 mg tabs
Metformin/sitagliptin – *Janumet* (Merck)	500/50, 1000/50 mg tabs
Metformin/saxagliptin – *Kombiglyze XR*	500/5, 1000/2.5, 1000/5 mg
(Bristol-Myers Squibb)	ER tabs

15. Once-daily dosing should be given with the evening meal.

cells, lowering serum glucose concentrations, without causing nausea or delaying gastric emptying.

***DPP-4 ENZYME INHIBITORS* – Sitagliptin** phosphate *(Januvia)*, an oral DPP-4 inhibitor, is FDA-approved for use as monotherapy or in combination with metformin, a sulfonylurea, pioglitazone or insulin in patients with type 2 diabetes.[19] Efficacy trials of sitagliptin have shown reductions in A1C concentrations of 0.6-0.8% more than with placebo.[20-22] Sitagliptin is available in a fixed-dose combination with metformin *(Janumet)*. It is also available in combination with simvastatin *(Juvisync)*.[50]

Saxagliptin *(Onglyza)* is FDA-approved for treatment of type 2 diabetes, alone or in combination with metformin, a sulfonylurea or pioglitazone, but not with insulin. It produces an average A1C reduction of 0.4-0.8% when compared with placebo.[23-25] Saxagliptin is available in a fixed-dose

Pregnancy Category[1]	Usual Daily Dosage
C	500 mg/15 mg PO bid[2,3]
C	1000 mg/15 mg PO once[2,4] 500 mg/1-2 mg PO bid-tid[2,7]
C	500 mg/2 mg PO bid[2,3]
C	
C	4 mg/4 mg PO bid 4 mg/30 mg PO once
B	500 mg/50 mg PO bid[2,3]
B	1000-2000 mg/5 mg PO once[2,15]

combination with extended-release metformin *(Kombiglyze XR)*; studies using saxagliptin with immediate-release metformin have shown additional reductions in A1C of 0.5-0.8% compared to either agent alone.[23-26]

Linagliptin *(Tradjenta)*, a third DPP-4 inhibitor, is approved by the FDA for treatment of type 2 diabetes, alone or in combination with metformin, a sulfonylurea or pioglitazone. In clinical trials, linagliptin has produced placebo-adjusted reductions in A1C of 0.5-0.7%.[27] Linagliptin is available in a fixed-dose combination with metformin *(Jentadueto)*. Unlike sitagliptin and saxagliptin, the dose of linagliptin does not need to be adjusted in patients with renal dysfunction.

Adverse Effects – DPP-4 inhibitors appear to be weight neutral.[20] The incidence of hypoglycemic events increases significantly when these drugs are added to a sulfonylurea.[21,24] The long-term safety of DPP-4 inhibitors is unknown; DPP-4 cleaves many other peptides besides the incretin hormones, including neuropeptides, cytokines and chemokines. Pancreatitis has been reported with sitagliptin and linagliptin, including hemorrhagic or necrotizing pancreatitis with sitagliptin. Hypersensitivity reactions including urticaria, angioedema, anaphylaxis, skin reactions such as Stevens-Johnson syndrome and hypersensitivity vasculitis have been reported with all DPP-4 inhibitors.

GLP-1 ANALOGS – **Exenatide** *(Byetta)* is FDA-approved for twice-daily subcutaneous injection in patients with type 2 diabetes who have not achieved adequate control with lifestyle modification, metformin, a sulfonylurea, pioglitazone or a combination of these drugs. Exenatide has an amino acid sequence similar to that of GLP-1, and in the presence of hyperglycemia acts to stimulate insulin secretion. In addition, it lowers serum glucagon concentrations, slows gastric emptying and increases satiety.[28] Trials have shown weight loss of 1.5-2.8 kg in patients treated with exenatide and a reduction in A1C of about 1.0%, compared to placebo.[29] Exenatide is also available in an extended-release formulation *(Bydureon)* given once weekly; it is not indicated for use with insulin. In trials, A1C decreased about 1.5% and weight loss was about 2.3 kg.[51]

Liraglutide *(Victoza)* is a GLP-1 receptor agonist given once daily by subcutaneous injection; like exenatide, it is not recommended for first-line therapy.[30] In clinical studies, liraglutide added to other drugs was either equal to or significantly better than oral comparators in reducing A1C; A1C reduction was typically 1.0-1.5%. Greater weight loss (up to a 2.8-kg difference) was seen in most studies, but not all.[31] Compared with exenatide, liraglutide has a greater effect on fasting glucose levels, but less effect on postprandial levels.

Adverse Effects – Nausea, vomiting and diarrhea have been the most common adverse effects of GLP-1 analogs; to help reduce nausea, the dose of either agent should be titrated up slowly as tolerated (typically over one week for liraglutide, one month for exenatide). Neither drug causes significant hypoglycemia, except in combination with a sulfonylurea; the dose of the sulfonylurea should be reduced when starting either drug. Because it slows gastric emptying, exenatide can decrease the rate and extent of absorption of other drugs; it should not be used in patients with gastroparesis. Acute pancreatitis has been reported with both agents. Thyroid C-cell carcinomas have been reported in rodents given liraglutide; thyroid C-cell hyperplasia has been reported in human clinical trials.

Renal insufficiency and acute renal failure have occurred with exenatide, and have usually been associated with nausea and vomiting in patients with pre-existing kidney disease or in those using other drugs with a potential for nephrotoxicity. Liraglutide can be used in patients with mild renal insufficiency.

COLESEVELAM — A bile-acid sequestrant used to lower LDL cholesterol, colesevelam *(Welchol)* is approved by the FDA as an adjunct to diet and exercise for the treatment of type 2 diabetes.[32] In patients taking metformin, a sulfonylurea or insulin, it has reduced A1C by about 0.5% more than placebo.[33] The mechanism is unclear. It is not recommended for monotherapy.

Adverse Effects – Colesevelam causes constipation, nausea and dyspepsia, increases serum triglyceride concentrations and interferes with absorption of other oral drugs.

BROMOCRIPTINE — A new formulation of the ergot-derived dopamine agonist bromocriptine *(Cycloset)* has been marginally effective in decreasing blood glucose levels in patients with type 2 diabetes.[34]

Adverse Effects – Nausea and vomiting have been the most common adverse effects and may make the drug difficult to tolerate. Fatigue, headache and dizziness can also occur.

SOME INSULIN PRODUCTS

	Formulation[1]
RAPID-ACTING	
Insulin aspart –	
Novolog (Novo Nordisk)	10 mL vial, 3 mL cartridge, 3 mL *FlexPen*[3]
Insulin lispro – *Humalog* (Lilly)	10 mL vial, 3 mL cartridge, 3 mL *KwikPen*[3]
Insulin glulisine – *Apidra* (Sanofi-Aventis)	10 mL vial, 3 mL cartridge,[4] 3 mL *Solostar*
REGULAR INSULIN	
Humulin R (Lilly)	10 mL vial[5]
Novolin R (Novo Nordisk)	10 mL vial, 3 mL *PenFill* cartridge, 3 mL Innolet
INTERMEDIATE-ACTING	
NPH	
Humulin N (Lilly)	10 mL vial, 3 mL *PenFill* cartridge
Novolin N (NovoNordisk)	10 mL vial, 3 mL *PenFill* cartridge, 3 mL *Innolet*
LONG-ACTING	
Insulin detemir –	
Levemir (Novo Nordisk)	10 mL vial, 3 mL cartridge, 3 mL *FlexPen*[3], 3 mL *Innolet*
Insulin glargine – *Lantus* (Sanofi-Aventis)	10 mL vial, 3 mL cartridge,[4] 3 mL *SoloStar* disposable device
PRE-MIXED	
Novolin 70/30 (Novo Nordisk) (70% NPH, human insulin isophane susp and 30% regular human insulin injection)	10 mL vial, 3 mL *PenFill* cartridge,[6] 3 mL *Innolet*

1. Cartridges are used with pen injectors.
2. FDA pregnancy categories: B = no evidence of risk in humans; C = risk cannot be ruled out.
3. Prefilled, disposable syringe.

Onset	Peak	Duration	Pregnancy Category[2]
10-30 min	30 min-3 hrs	3-5 hrs	
			B
			B
			C
30-60 min	2½-5 hrs	4-12 hrs	
			B
			B
1-2 hrs	4-8 hrs	10-20 hrs	
			B
			B
1-4 hrs	relatively flat	12-20 hrs	C
1-4 hrs	no peak	22-24 hrs	C
30-60 min	2-12 hrs	18-24 hrs	B

4. For use with *OptiClick* device.
5. Also available in a concentrated formula with 500 units per mL.
6. For use with *NovoPen 4* or *Novopen Jr.*

Continued on next page.

SOME INSULIN PRODUCTS (continued)

	Formulation[1]
PRE-MIXED (continued)	
Novolog Mix 70/30 (Novo Nordisk) (70% insulin aspart protamine susp and 30% insulin aspart injection)	10 mL vial, 3 mL *FlexPen*
Humalog Mix 75/25 (Lilly) (75% insulin lispro protamine susp and 25% insulin lispro injection)	10 mL vial, 3 mL *Pen*, 3 mL *KwikPen*

PRAMLINTIDE *(Symlin)* is an amylinomimetic agent that is injected subcutaneously before meals.[35] It has been approved for use in patients with type 1 or type 2 diabetes on prandial insulin who have not been able to achieve blood glucose targets. Pramlintide acts by slowing gastric emptying, increasing satiety and suppressing postprandial plasma glucagon and hepatic glucose production. Patients with type 2 diabetes start pramlintide at 60 mcg before meals, and then increase to 120 mcg as tolerated. Its major effect seems to be reducing postprandial glucose excursions and promoting weight loss; the effect on A1C is modest (about a 0.3-0.6% decrease).[36]

Adverse Effects – Nausea, vomiting, anorexia and headache can occur. Pramlintide may delay or decrease absorption of oral drugs taken at the same time. The drug should not be used in patients with gastroparesis or in those taking other drugs that may alter gastrointestinal motility. Used in combination with insulin, pramlintide has been associated with severe hypoglycemia. A reduction in short-acting insulin dosages, including pre-mixed insulins, of 50% with initiation of pramlintide therapy and frequent (including postprandial) glucose monitoring are recommended.

Onset	Peak	Duration	Pregnancy Category[2]
10-20 min	1-4 hrs	18-24 hrs	B
10-30 min	1-6½ hrs	14-24 hrs	B

REGULAR AND RAPID-ACTING INSULINS — Rapid-acting insulin analogs have a more rapid onset and shorter duration of action than regular insulin. In general, **insulin lispro**, **insulin aspart** and **insulin glulisine** are slightly more effective than regular insulin in decreasing A1C, with less hypoglycemia.[37-39]

Adverse Effects – With all insulins, the greatest risk is hypoglycemia. The risk with the rapid-acting insulin analogs is less than with regular insulin.

LONGER-ACTING INSULINS — An intermediate-acting insulin such as **NPH** can be used in combination with regular and rapid-acting insulins. Alternatively, patients can use pre-mixed combinations. While these formulations simplify administration of insulin, titration of dose is more difficult and hypoglycemia may be more frequent than with individual insulins.

Insulin glargine,[40] a recombinant DNA analog of human insulin, forms microprecipitates in subcutaneous tissue, prolonging its duration of action to a mean of about 24 hours. It has a less pronounced peak of action than NPH insulin and does not show differing rates of absorption when injected at various sites.

Insulin detemir has both delayed absorption from subcutaneous tissue and, due to reversible binding to albumin, delayed clearance from the circulation. Both glargine and detemir are equivalent to NPH in lowering A1C, but cause less nocturnal hypoglycemia.[41,42] Insulin detemir may be more effective when used twice daily; after 12 hours, its effectiveness appears to decrease.

Adverse Effects – All insulins, including long-acting formulations, can cause hypoglycemia and weight gain. In a comparative trial, detemir caused more injection site reactions than glargine (4.5% vs. 1.4%).[43] The long-term safety of NPH insulin has been established. *In vitro*, insulin glargine has higher affinity for the insulin-like growth factor (IGF-1) receptor than other insulins. Some observational studies have found an increased risk of cancer in patients using glargine alone; other studies have found either no increased risk or a trend towards a decreased risk of cancer when glargine was used with other insulins.[44]

ADDITION OF INSULIN — When insulin is added to oral agents, it is usually given either in the evening or at bedtime. In general, added insulin can be started with 10 units (or 0.2-0.5 units/kg) of a pre-mixed combination at dinnertime, or NPH, detemir or glargine at bedtime. The dose can then be increased to achieve fasting plasma glucose concentrations between 70-130 mg/dL.

Biphasic (pre-mixed) insulin (30% rapid-acting insulin aspart and 70% intermediate-acting protaminated insulin aspart) given twice daily, prandial insulin given before meals three times daily, and basal insulin (bedtime or twice-daily insulin detemir) were compared as initial insulin therapy in 708 patients with type 2 diabetes and suboptimal glucose control (mean A1C 8.5%) on maximum tolerated doses of metformin and a sulfonylurea. After 3 years, all regimens achieved similar A1C levels

(6.8-7.1%) with the most weight gain and hypoglycemia in the prandial group and the least in the basal group. In all groups, <50% of patients achieved A1C levels <6.5%.[45]

GLYCEMIC THERAPY GOALS — The goal of drug therapy for type 2 diabetes is achieving and maintaining a near-normal A1C concentration without inducing hypoglycemia; the target is generally an A1C of $\leq$7.0%. Treating to this target has clearly been shown to prevent the microvascular complications of retinopathy and nephropathy, but whether it prevents macrovascular outcomes is unclear. Three large trials have found no decrease in macrovascular events with intensive glucose control.[46-48] One of these trials (the ACCORD trial) in about 10,000 patients with type 2 diabetes at high-risk for cardiovascular disease found that patients intensively treated with anti-hyperglycemic drugs, including frequent use of TZDs and insulin with an A1C target of 6.0%, did not significantly reduce the incidence of major cardiovascular events (the primary endpoint) over a period of 3.5 years and increased all-cause mortality compared to patients treated with an A1C target of 7.0-7.9%.[46] Levels near 7.0% may be prudent in older patients with a long duration of type 2 diabetes, and in those with underlying cardiovascular disease, frequent hypoglycemia or multiple diabetes-related complications or co-morbidities.[49]

1. DM Nathan et al. Medical management of hyperglycemia in type 2 diabetes: a consensus algorithm for the initiation and adjustment of therapy: a consensus statement of the American Diabetes Association and the European Association for the Study of Diabetes. Diabetes Care 2009; 32:193.
2. RR Holman et al. 10-year follow-up of intensive glucose control in type 2 diabetes. N Engl J Med 2008; 359:1577.
3. J deJager et al. Long term treatment with metformin in patients with type 2 diabetes and risk of vitamin B-12 deficiency: randomized placebo controlled trial. BMJ 2010; 340:c2181.
4. SE Inzucchi et al. Metformin in heart failure. Diabetes Care 2007; 30:e129.
5. SE Kahn et al. Glycemic durability of rosiglitazone, metformin, or glyburide monotherapy (The ADOPT Study Group). N Engl J Med 2006; 355:2427.
6. MC Riddle. More reasons to say goodbye to glyburide. J Clin Endocrinol Metab 2010; 95:4867.
7. M Zeller et al. Impact of type of preadmission sulfonylureas on mortality and cardiovascular outcomes in diabetic patients with acute myocardial infarction. J Clin Endocrinol Metab 2010; 95:4993.

Drugs for Type 2 Diabetes

8. Repaglinide for type 2 diabetes mellitus. Med Lett Drugs Ther 1998; 40:55.
9. Nateglinide for type 2 diabetes. Med Lett Drugs Ther 2001; 43:29.
10. S Bolen et al. Systematic review: comparative effectiveness and safety of oral medications for type 2 diabetes mellitus. Ann Intern Med 2007; 147:386.
11. Rosiglitazone (Avandia) revisited. Med Lett Drugs Ther 2010; 52:17.
12. SE Nissen and K Wolski. Effect of rosiglitazone on the risk of myocardial infarction and death from cardiovascular causes. N Engl J Med 2007; 356:2457.
13. RM Lago et al. Congestive heart failure and cardiovascular death in patients with prediabetes and type 2 diabetes given thiazolidinediones: a meta-analysis of randomized clinical trials. Lancet 2007; 370:1129.
14. DJ Graham et al. Risk of acute myocardial infarction, stroke, heart failure and death in elderly Medicare patients treated with rosiglitazone or pioglitazone. JAMA 2010; 304:411.
15. DN Juurlink et al. Adverse cardiovascular events during treatment with pioglitazone and rosiglitazone: population based cohort study. BMJ 2009; 339:b2942.
16. Updated Risk Evaluation and Mitigation Strategy (REMS) to restrict access to rosiglitazone-containing medicines including Avandia, Avandamet and Avandryl. Available at http://www.fda.gov/Drugs/Drug Safety/ucm255005.htm. Accessed June 6, 2011.
17. YK Loke et al. Long-term use of thiazolidinediones and fractures in type 2 diabetes: a meta-analysis. CMAJ 2009; 180:32.
18. FDA Drug Safety Communication. Update to ongoing safety review of Actos (pioglitazone) and increased risk of bladder cancer. Available at www.fda.gov/Drugs/DrugSafety/ucm226214.htm. Accessed June 29, 2011.
19. Sitagliptin (Januvia) for type 2 diabetes. Med Lett Drugs Ther 2007; 49:1.
20. BJ Goldstein et al. Effect of initial combination therapy with sitagliptin, a dipeptidyl peptidase-4 inhibitor, and metformin on glycemic control in patients with type 2 diabetes. Diabetes Care 2007; 30:1979.
21. K Hermansen et al. Efficacy and safety of the dipeptidyl peptidase-4 inhibitor, sitagliptin, in patients with type 2 diabetes mellitus inadequately controlled on glimepiride alone or on glimepiride and metformin. Diabetes Obes Metab 2007; 9:733.
22. P Aschner et al. Efficacy and safety of monotherapy of sitagliptin compared with metformin in patients with type 2 diabetes. Diabetes Obes Metab 2010; 12:252.
23. RA DeFronzo et al. The efficacy and safety of saxagliptin when added to metformin therapy in patients with inadequately controlled type 2 diabetes with metformin alone. Diabetes Care 2009; 32:1649.
24. AR Chacra et al. Saxagliptin added to a submaximal dose of sulphonylurea improves glycaemic control compared with uptitration of sulphonylurea in patients with type 2 diabetes: a randomized controlled trial. Int J Clin Pract 2009; 63:1395.
25. P Hollander et al. Saxagliptin added to thiazolidinedione improves glycemic control in patients with type 2 diabetes and inadequate control on thiazolidinedione alone. J Clin Endocrinol Metab 2009; 94:4810.
26. M Jadzinsky et al. Saxagliptin given in combination with metformin as initial therapy improves glycaemic control in patients with type 2 diabetes compared with either monotherapy: a randomized controlled trial. Diabetes Obes Metab 2009; 11:611.

27. Linagliptin (Tradjenta) – a new DPP-4 inhibitor for type 2 diabetes. Med Lett Drugs Ther 2011; 53:49.
28. Exenatide (Byetta) for type 2 diabetes. Med Lett Drugs Ther 2005; 47:45.
29. RE Amori et al. Efficacy and safety of incretin therapy in type 2 diabetes: systematic review and meta-analysis. JAMA 2007; 298:194.
30. Liraglutide (Victoza) for type 2 diabetes. Med Lett Drugs Ther 2010; 52:25.
31. JA Davidson et al. Mild renal impairment has no effect on the efficacy and safety of liraglutide. Endocr Pract 2010; Dec 6:1-31. Epub.
32. A new indication for colesevelam (Welchol). Med Lett Drugs Ther 2008; 50:33.
33. J Rosenstock et al. Initial combination therapy with metformin and colesevelam for achievement of glycemic and lipid goals in early type 2 diabetes. Endocr Pract 2010; 16:629.
34. Bromocriptine (Cycloset) for type 2 diabetes. Med Lett Drugs Ther 2010; 52:97.
35. Pramlintide (Symlin) for diabetes. Med Lett Drugs Ther 2005; 47:43.
36. RE Ratner et al. Amylin replacement with pramlintide as an adjunct to insulin therapy improves long-term glycaemic and weight control in type 1 diabetes mellitus: a 1-year, randomized controlled trial. Diabet Med 2004; 21:1204.
37. SR Singh et al. Efficacy and safety of insulin analogs for the management of diabetes mellitus: a meta-analysis. CMAJ 2009; 180:385.
38. Rapid-acting insulin analogs. Med Lett Drugs Ther 2009; 51:98.
39. Insulin glulisine (Apidra), a new rapid-acting insulin. Med Lett Drugs Ther 2006; 48:33.
40. Insulin glargine (Lantus), a new long-acting insulin. Med Lett Drugs Ther 2001; 43:65.
41. Insulin detemir (Levemir), a new long-acting insulin. Med Lett Drugs Ther 2006; 48:54.
42. K Hermansen et al. A 26-week, randomized, parallel, treat-to-target trial comparing insulin detemir with NPH insulin as add-on therapy to oral glucose-lowering drugs in insulin-naive people with type 2 diabetes. Diabetes Care 2006; 29:1269.
43. J Rosenstock et al. A randomized, 52-week, treat-to-target trial comparing insulin detemir with insulin glargine when administered as add-on to glucose-lowering drugs in insulin naive people with type 2 diabetes. Diabetologia 2008; 51:408.
44. Insulin glargine (Lantus) and cancer risk. Med Lett Drugs Ther 2009; 51:67.
45. RR Holman et al. Three-year efficacy of complex insulin regimens in type 2 diabetes. N Engl J Med 2009; 361:1736.
46. ACCORD study group. Long-term effects of intensive glucose lowering on cardiovascular outcomes. N Engl J Med 2011; 364:818.
47. The ADVANCE Collaborative Group. Intensive blood glucose control and vascular outcomes in patients with type 2 diabetes. N Engl J Med 2008; 358:2560.
48. W Duckworth et al. Glucose control and vascular complications in veterans with type 2 diabetes. N Engl J Med 2009; 360:129.
49. J Skyler et al. Intensive glycemic control and the prevention of cardiovascular events: implications of the ACCORD, ADVANCE and the VA diabetes trials: a position statement of the American Diabetes Association and a scientific statement of the American College of Cardiology Foundation and the American Heart Association. Circulation 2009; 119:351.
50. Sitagliptin and simvastatin (Juvisync). Med Lett Drugs Ther 2011; 53:89.
51. Extended-release exenatide (Bydureon) for type 2 diabetes. Med Lett Drugs Ther 2012; 54:21.

DRUGS FOR
Hypertension

Original publication date – January 2012 (revised March 2012)

RECOMMENDATIONS: In many patients, a thiazide diuretic remains a reasonable choice for initial treatment of hypertension. Chlorthalidone appears to be more effective than hydrochlorothiazide (HCTZ) in lowering blood pressure (BP) and has been shown to be as effective as a calcium channel blocker or an angiotensin-converting enzyme (ACE) inhibitor in preventing cardiovascular events in hypertensive patients with coronary risk factors. An ACE inhibitor, an angiotensin receptor blocker (ARB) or a calcium channel blocker would also be a good choice for initial therapy. In black patients, diuretics and calcium channel blockers are more effective than ACE inhibitors or ARBs. The choice of antihypertensive agents for some patients may be dictated by concomitant conditions and their treatment.

Generally, if the first drug chosen is ineffective, a drug with a different mechanism of action should be substituted or added. The addition of a second drug with a different mechanism of action is usually more effective in decreasing BP than raising the dose of the first drug and often allows for use of lower doses of both drugs, improving tolerability. If an ACE inhibitor or an ARB was used initially, it would be reasonable to add a diuretic such as chlorthalidone. For patients with resistant hypertension, adding spironolactone can be helpful.

Most patients eventually require 2 or more drugs to achieve their blood pressure goals. When baseline BP is >20/10 mm Hg above goal, many experts would begin therapy with 2 drugs. The use of fixed-dose combinations may facilitate adherence.

Drugs available in the US for treatment of chronic hypertension, with their dosages and adverse effects, are listed in the tables that begin on page 140. Combination products are listed on page 160. Drugs for treatment of hypertensive emergencies are not discussed here. They were reviewed previously.[1,2]

DIURETICS

Thiazide-type diuretics are the first-line therapy for many patients with hypertension. **Chlorthalidone** and **hydrochlorothiazide (HCTZ)** are often prescribed at a dose of 12.5-25 mg once daily. Chlorthalidone is, however, 1.5-2 times more potent than HCTZ and has a longer duration of action that persists throughout the nighttime hours.[3] In a study that measured 24-hour ambulatory blood pressure (BP), chlorthalidone 25 mg was more effective than HCTZ 50 mg in lowering BP.[4]

HCTZ is by far the most widely used thiazide-type diuretic, even though no outcomes data are available for the most commonly used doses; studies documenting the effectiveness of HCTZ in reducing clinical outcomes used doses of $\geq$25 mg/day.[5] Most studies that have shown outcome benefits of thiazide-type diuretics have used chlorthalidone. In a double-blind, randomized controlled trial (ALLHAT) in more than 30,000 men and women $\geq$55 years old with hypertension and at least one risk factor for coronary heart disease, chlorthalidone 12.5-25 mg/day was as effective as the calcium channel blocker amlodipine or the angiotensin-converting enzyme (ACE) inhibitor lisinopril in preventing fatal coronary heart disease or nonfatal myocardial infarction. At the end of 5 years, about 40% of patients had required at least one additional drug to achieve the BP goal of 140/90 mm Hg.[6,7]

The number of fixed-dose combination products containing chlorthalidone as the diuretic is smaller than the number containing HCTZ. A fixed-dose combination of chlorthalidone and azilsartan *(Edarbyclor)* has recently become available.[8]

Metolazone may be effective in patients with impaired renal function when the other thiazides are not, but data are lacking. **Indapamide** with or without the ACE inhibitor perindopril was effective in one study in elderly patients ($\geq$80 years old) in reducing death from stroke or any cause.[9]

Loop diuretics such as **furosemide** are more effective than thiazides in lowering BP in patients with moderate to severe renal insufficiency (CrCl <30 mL/min). In patients with normal renal function, they are less effective than thiazides for treatment of hypertension. **Ethacrynic acid** can be used in patients allergic to sulfonamides (thiazide and other loop diuretics contain sulfonamide moieties).

Potassium-sparing agents such as **amiloride** and **triamterene** are generally used with other diuretics to prevent or correct hypokalemia. These drugs can cause hyperkalemia, particularly in patients with renal impairment and in those taking ACE inhibitors, angiotensin receptor blockers (ARBs), beta blockers or direct renin inhibitors.

Spironolactone, a mineralocorticoid receptor antagonist also used as a potassium-sparing diuretic, has been effective as an add-on in patients with resistant hypertension.[10] **Eplerenone**, a selective mineralocorticoid receptor antagonist,[11] is less likely than higher doses of spironolactone to cause gynecomastia. Aldosterone antagonism may provide cardiovascular benefits beyond minimizing hypokalemia.[12] Both spironolactone and eplerenone have been shown to reduce mortality in patients with heart failure when added to standard therapy.[13]

Drugs for Hypertension

DIURETICS[1]

Drug	Some Oral Formulations	Usual Daily Maintenance Dosage
THIAZIDE-TYPE		
Chlorthalidone –		12.5-50 mg once
generic	25, 50 mg tabs	
Thalitone (Monarch)	15 mg tabs	
Chlorothiazide –		125-500 mg once
generic	250, 500 mg tabs	
Diuril (Salix)	250 mg/5mL susp	
Hydrochlorothiazide –		12.5-50 mg once
generic[4]	12.5 mg caps;	
	12.5, 25, 50 mg tabs	
Microzide (Watson)	12.5 mg caps	
Indapamide –	1.25, 2.5 mg tabs	1.25-5 mg once
generic[4]		
Metolazone – generic	2.5, 5, 10 mg tabs	1.25-5 mg once
Zaroxolyn (UCB Pharma)		
LOOP		
Bumetanide – generic[4]	0.5, 1, 2 mg tabs	0.5-2 mg in 2 doses
Ethacrynic acid –	25 mg tabs	25-100 mg in
Edecrin (Aton Pharma)		2 or 3 doses
Furosemide – generic[4]	20, 40, 80 mg tabs;	20-320 mg in
	10 mg/mL, 40 mg/5 mL soln	2 doses
Lasix (Sanofi)	20, 40, 80 mg tabs	
Torsemide – generic	5, 10, 20, 100 mg tabs	5-20 mg in
Demadex (Meda)		1 or 2 doses

1. Diuretics are not recommended for treatment of gestational hypertension.
2. FDA pregnancy categories: A = controlled studies show no risk; B = no evidence of risk; C = risk cannot be ruled out; D = positive evidence of risk; X = contraindicated in pregnancy

Pregnancy Category[2]	Frequent or Severe Adverse Effects[3]
B	
C	
B	Hyperuricemia, hypokalemia, hypomagnesemia, hyperglycemia, hyponatremia, hypercalcemia, hypercholesterolemia, hyper-triglyceridemia, pancreatitis, rash and other allergic reactions, sexual dysfunction in men, photosensitivity reactions
B	
B	
C	
B	Dehydration, circulatory collapse, hypokalemia, hyponatremia, hypomagnesemia, hyperglycemia, metabolic alkalosis, hyperuricemia, blood dyscrasias, rash, hypercholesterolemia, hypertriglyceridemia
C	
B	

3. In addition to the adverse effects listed, antihypertensive drugs may interact adversely with other drugs.
4. A 30-day supply of some strengths is available for $4 at some discount pharmacies.

Continued on next page.

DIURETICS[1] (continued)

Drug	Some Oral Formulations	Usual Daily Maintenance Dosage
POTASSIUM-SPARING		
Amiloride – generic	5 mg tabs	5-10 mg in
Midamor (Paddock)		1 or 2 doses
Eplerenone – generic	25, 50 mg tabs	25-100 mg in
Inspra (Pfizer)		1 or 2 doses
Spironolactone – generic[4]	25, 50, 100 mg tabs	12.5-100 mg in
Aldactone (Pfizer)		1 or 2 doses
Triamterene –		50-150 mg in
Dyrenium (WellSpring)	50, 100 mg caps	1 or 2 doses

ANGIOTENSIN-CONVERTING ENZYME (ACE) INHIBITORS

ACE inhibitors are effective in treating hypertension and are well tolerated. They are less effective in black patients and others with low-renin
hypertension, unless combined with a thiazide diuretic or calcium channel
blocker. ACE inhibitors have been shown to prolong survival in patients
with heart failure or left ventricular dysfunction after a myocardial infarction, reduce mortality in patients without heart failure or left ventricular
dysfunction who are at high risk for cardiovascular events, and reduce
proteinuria in patients with either diabetic or non-diabetic nephropathy.[14]
In an open-label trial (ANBP2) among more than 6000 mostly white
patients with a low incidence of diabetes, ACE inhibitor-treated male
patients had an 11% lower incidence of cardiovascular events or all-cause
mortality than those treated with various doses of thiazide diuretics,
despite similar reductions in BP.[15] However, among 15,700 mostly white
patients in the double-blind ALLHAT study, treatment of hypertension
with an ACE inhibitor did not improve cardiovascular outcomes compared to chlorthalidone 12.5-25 mg. In black hypertensive participants in

Pregnancy Category[2]	Frequent or Severe Adverse Effects[3]
B	Hyperkalemia, GI disturbances, rash, headache
B	Hyperkalemia, hyponatremia
D	Hyperkalemia, hyponatremia, mastodynia, gynecomastia, menstrual abnormalities, GI disturbances, rash
C	Hyperkalemia, GI disturbances, nephrolithiasis

ALLHAT, the ACE inhibitor regimen was less effective than the diuretic in lowering BP and less effective in reducing the incidence of stroke and cardiovascular events.[6]

ANGIOTENSIN RECEPTOR BLOCKERS (ARBs)

ARBs are as effective as ACE inhibitors in lowering BP, and appear to be equally reno- and cardioprotective, with fewer adverse effects. Like ACE inhibitors, they are less effective in black patients and others with low-renin hypertension, unless combined with a thiazide diuretic or calcium channel blocker. **Irbesartan** treatment delayed development of overt diabetic nephropathy in hypertensive patients with type 2 diabetes.[16] In diabetic patients who already had overt nephropathy, **irbesartan** and **losartan** slowed progression of the renal disease.[17,18] In patients with hypertension and left ventricular hypertrophy, with or without diabetes (LIFE), losartan was more effective in decreasing stroke, than the beta blocker atenolol, but not in black patients.[19] The ARBs **valsartan** and **candesartan** have been shown to slow disease progression in patients with chronic heart failure

Drugs for Hypertension

RENIN-ANGIOTENSIN SYSTEM INHIBITORS

Drug	Some Oral Formulations	Usual Daily Maintenance Dosage
ANGIOTENSIN-CONVERTING ENZYMES (ACE) INHIBITORS		
Benazepril – generic[4]	5, 10, 20, 40 mg tabs	10-80 mg in
Lotensin (Novartis)		1 or 2 doses
Captopril – generic[4]	12.5, 25, 50, 100 mg tabs	12.5-150 mg in
Capoten (Par)		2 or 3 doses
Enalapril – generic[4]	2.5, 5, 10, 20 mg tabs	2.5-40 mg in
Vasotec (Valeant)		1-2 doses
Fosinopril – generic	10, 20, 40 mg tabs	10-80 mg in
Monopril (BMS)		1 or 2 doses
Lisinopril – generic[4]	2.5, 5, 10, 20, 30, 40 mg tabs	5-40 mg once
Prinivil (Merck)		
Zestril[5] (AstraZeneca)		
Moexipril – generic	7.5, 15 mg tabs	7.5-30 mg in
Univasc (UCB Pharma)		1 or 2 doses
Perindopril – generic	2, 4, 8 mg tabs	4-8 mg in
Aceon (Abbott)		1 or 2 doses
Quinapril – generic	5, 10, 20, 40 mg tabs	5-80 mg in
Accupril (Pfizer)		1 or 2 doses
Ramipril – generic	1.25, 2.5, 5, 10 mg caps	1.25-20 mg in
Altace (King)		1 or 2 doses
Trandolapril – generic	1, 2, 4 mg tabs	1-8 mg in
Mavik (Abbott)		1 or 2 doses

1. ACE inhibitors, ARBs and aliskiren are rated category C during the first trimester and category D during the second and third trimesters. Drugs that act on the renin-angiotensin system can cause fetal and neonatal morbidity and death.
2. FDA pregnancy categories: A = controlled studies show no risk; B = no evidence of risk; C = risk cannot be ruled out; D = positive evidence of risk; X = contraindicated in pregnancy

Pregnancy Category[1,2]	Frequent or Severe Adverse Effects[3]
D	
C/D	
C/D	
C/D	Cough, hypotension (particularly with diuretic use or volume depletion), rash, acute renal failure in patients with bilateral
C/D	renal artery stenosis or stenosis of the artery to a solitary kidney, angioedema, hyperkalemia (particularly if also taking potassium supplements or potassium-sparing diuretics), mild-
C/D	to-moderate loss of taste, hepatotoxicity, pancreatitis, blood dyscrasias and renal damage (particularly in patients with
D	renal dysfunction), increased fetal malformations and mortality with use in pregnancy
C/D	
C/D	
C/D	

3. In addition to the adverse effects listed, antihypertensive drugs may interact adversely with other drugs.
4. A 30-day supply of some strengths is available for $4 at some discount pharmacies.
5. Not available as 2.5 or 30 mg tablets.

Continued on next page.

Drugs for Hypertension

RENIN-ANGIOTENSIN SYSTEM INHIBITORS (continued)

Drug	Some Oral Formulations	Usual Daily Maintenance Dosage
ANGIOTENSIN RECEPTOR BLOCKERS (ARBs)		
Azilsartan – *Edarbi* (Takeda)	40, 80 mg tabs	80 mg once
Candesartan – *Atacand* (AstraZeneca)	4, 8, 16, 32 mg tabs	8-32 mg once
Eprosartan – *Teveten* (Abbott)	400, 600 mg tabs	400-800 mg in 1 or 2 doses
Irbesartan – *Avapro* (BMS/Sanofi)	75, 150, 300 mg tabs	150-300 mg once
Losartan – generic *Cozaar* (Merck)	25, 50, 100 mg tabs	25-100 mg in 1 or 2 doses
Olmesartan – *Benicar* (Daiichi Sankyo)	5, 20, 40 mg tabs	20-40 mg once
Telmisartan – *Micardis* (Boehringer Ingelheim)	20, 40, 80 mg tabs	40-80 mg once
Valsartan – *Diovan* (Novartis)	40, 80, 160, 320 mg tabs	80-320 mg once
DIRECT RENIN INHIBITOR (DRI)		
Aliskiren – *Tekturna* (Novartis)	150, 300 mg tabs	150-300 mg once

(Val-HeFT, VALIANT, CHARM).[20-22] **Telmisartan** was as effective as the ACE inhibitor ramipril in preventing cardiovascular events in high-risk hypertensive patients with diabetes or vascular disease (ONTARGET); the combination of an ACE inhibitor and an ARB provided no additional benefit on cardiovascular or renal outcomes compared to either agent alone, but was more effective in lowering BP.[23]

DIRECT RENIN INHIBITOR

Aliskiren, a direct renin inhibitor (DRI), is FDA-approved alone or in combination with other antihypertensive drugs for treatment of hyperten-

Pregnancy Category[1,2]	Frequent or Severe Adverse Effects[3]
C/D	
C/D	
C/D	Similar to ACE inhibitors, including increased fetal mortality with use in pregnancy, but do not cause cough and only rarely cause angioedema, loss of taste and hepatotoxicity; rarely rhabdomyolysis
C/D	
C/D	
C/D	
D	
C/D	Same as ARBs, but can also cause GI effects such as diarrhea

sion.[24] Whether aliskiren offers any advantage over ACE inhibitors or ARBs remains to be determined, and no outcomes data are available for aliskiren. In an 8-week study, concurrent use of aliskiren and the ARB valsartan was significantly more effective in lowering BP than either agent alone.[25] However, a randomized trial evaluating the addition of an ACE inhibitor or an ARB to aliskiren in patients with type 2 diabetes and renal impairment was terminated prematurely due to an increase in adverse cardiovascular and renal events with the combination.[40]

Continued on page 152

Drugs for Hypertension

CALCIUM CHANNEL BLOCKERS

Drug	Some Oral Formulations	Usual Daily Maintenance Dosage
DIHYDROPYRIDINES		
Amlodipine[3] – generic	2.5, 5, 10 mg tabs	2.5-10 mg once
Norvasc (Pfizer)		
Felodipine – generic	2.5, 5, 10 mg ER tabs	2.5-10 mg once
Plendil (AstraZeneca)		
Isradipine – generic	2.5, 5 mg caps	5-10 mg in 2 doses
extended-release		
DynaCirc CR (GSK)	5, 10 mg ER tabs	5-10 mg once
Nicardipine – generic	20, 30 mg caps	60-120 mg in 3 doses
extended-release	30, 60 mg ER caps	60-120 mg in 2 doses
Cardene SR (EKR)		
Nifedipine –		
extended-release generic	30, 60, 90 mg ER tabs	30-90 mg once
Adalat CC (Bayer)		
Procardia XL (Pfizer)		
Nisoldipine – generic	8.5, 17, 20, 25.5, 30, 34, 40 mg ER tabs	17-40 mg once
Sular (Shionogi)	8.5, 17, 25.5, 34 mg ER tabs	17-34 mg once

1. FDA pregnancy categories: A = controlled studies show no risk; B = no evidence of risk; C = risk cannot be ruled out; D = positive evidence of risk; X = contraindicated in pregnancy
2. In addition to the adverse effects listed, antihypertensive drugs may interact adversely with other drugs.

148

Pregnancy Category[1]	Frequent or Severe Adverse Effects[2]
C	
C	
C	
C	
	Dizziness, headache, peripheral edema (more than with verapamil and diltiazem, more common in women), flushing, tachycardia, rash, gingival hyperplasia
C	
C	

3. Amlodipine is also available in combination with atorvastatin (*Caduet* – Pfizer).

Continued on next page.

CALCIUM CHANNEL BLOCKERS (continued)

Drug	Some Oral Formulations	Usual Daily Maintenance Dosage
NON-DIHYDROPYRIDINES		
Diltiazem[4]		
generic (extended-release)	120, 180, 240, 300,	120-540 mg once
Cardizem LA (Abbott)	360, 420 mg ER tabs	
generic (sustained-release)	120, 180, 240, 300, 360	120-540 mg once
Taztia XT[5] (Watson)	mg ER caps	
Tiazac[6] (Forest)		
generic (continuous-delivery)	120, 180, 240, 300,	120-360 mg once
Cardizem CD (Valeant)	360 mg ER caps	
Cartia XT[7] (Watson)		
Dilt-CD[7] (Apotex)		
Verapamil (extended-release)[4]		
generic (tabs)	120, 180, 240 mg ER tabs	120-480 mg
generic (caps)	120, 180, 240, 360 mg	in 1 or 2 doses
	ER caps	
Calan SR (Pfizer)	120, 180, 240 mg ER tabs	
Isoptin SR (Ranbaxy)	120, 180, 240 mg ER tabs	
extended-release (once/day)		
Covera-HS (Pfizer)	180, 240 mg ER tabs	180-540 mg once
Verelan (Elan)	120, 180, 240, 360 mg	120-480 mg once
	ER caps	
Verelan PM (Elan)	100, 200, 300 mg	100-400 mg once
	ER caps	

4. A 30-day supply of some strengths is available for $4 at some discount pharmacies.
5. *Diltia XT* and *Dilacor XR* (both manufactured by Watson) are also ER capsules (available in 120, 180, 240 mg ER capsules).

Pregnancy Category[1]	Frequent or Severe Adverse Effects[2]
C	
C	Dizziness, headache, edema, constipation (especially verapamil), AV block, bradycardia, heart failure, lupus-like rash with diltiazem

6. Also available in 420 mg ER caps.
7. Not available in 360 mg ER caps.

CALCIUM CHANNEL BLOCKERS

Calcium channel blockers are a structurally and functionally heterogeneous class of drugs. They all cause vasodilatation, which decreases peripheral resistance. The cardiac response to decreased vascular resistance is variable; with some dihydropyridines (**felodipine**, **nicardipine**, **nisoldipine** and immediate-release **nifedipine**), an initial reflex tachycardia usually occurs, but **isradipine**, sustained-release **nifedipine** and **amlodipine** generally cause little increase in heart rate. The non-dihydropyridines **verapamil** and **diltiazem** slow heart rate, can affect atrioventricular (AV) conduction and should be used with caution in patients also taking a beta blocker.

In one meta-analysis, the risk of heart failure was higher in patients treated with calcium channel blockers compared to those treated with ACE inhibitors, beta blockers or diuretics.[26] One large double-blind trial (VALUE Trial) in more than 15,000 high-risk patients found similar rates of cardiovascular events with amlodipine and the ARB valsartan.[27] In one large outcomes trial, a combination of the ACE inhibitor benazepril with the calcium channel blocker amlodipine was more effective in preventing adverse cardiovascular outcomes than benazepril with HCTZ 12.5-25 mg.[28]

BETA-ADRENERGIC BLOCKERS

A beta blocker may be a good choice for treatment of hypertension in patients with another indication for a beta blocker, such as migraine, angina pectoris, myocardial infarction or heart failure. In other high-risk patients, large cardiovascular outcome trials have found a beta blocker less effective in preventing cardiovascular events (especially stroke) than an ACE inhibitor, an ARB, a calcium channel blocker or a diuretic.[29,30] Two guideline panels have recommended not using a beta blocker for initial therapy of hypertension.[31,32] Like ACE inhibitors and ARBs, beta blockers are less effective in black patients.

Pindolol, **acebutolol**, **penbutolol** and **carteolol** have intrinsic sympatho-mimetic activity (ISA). Beta blockers without ISA are preferred in patients with angina or a history of myocardial infarction.

Labetalol combines beta blockade with alpha-adrenergic receptor block-ade. **Carvedilol** is another beta blocker with alpha-blocking properties; compared to metoprolol, it is less likely to interfere with glycemic con-trol in patients with type 2 diabetes and hypertension.[33] **Nebivolol** does not have alpha-blocking properties but does have nitric-oxide-mediated vasodilating activity.[34]

ALPHA-ADRENERGIC BLOCKERS

Prazosin, **terazosin** and **doxazosin** cause less tachycardia than direct vasodilators (hydralazine, minoxidil), but more frequent postural hypoten-sion, especially after the first dose. Treatment of essential hypertension with doxazosin has been associated with an increased incidence of heart failure, stroke and combined cardiovascular disease compared to treat-ment with a diuretic (ALLHAT). Alpha-blockers provide symptomatic relief from prostatism in men, but may cause stress incontinence in women and postural hypotension in elderly patients.

CENTRAL ALPHA-ADRENERGIC AGONISTS

Drugs such as **clonidine**, **guanfacine** and **methyldopa** decrease sym-pathetic outflow, but do not inhibit reflex responses as completely as sympatholytic drugs that act peripherally. They do, however, frequently cause sedation, dry mouth and erectile dysfunction. Clonidine is often used for treatment of hypertensive urgencies. Due to its short half-life (~7 hours), it must be taken 2 to 3 times a day for adequate long-term management of chronic hypertension. Once daily guanfacine (half-life ~17 hours) is more convenient for treatment of chronic hypertension; at doses of 1 mg, which provide all or most of the drug's blood pressure-lowering effect, it is generally well tolerated.

Drugs for Hypertension

BETA-ADRENERGIC BLOCKERS

Drug	Some Oral Formulations	Usual Daily Maintenance Dosage
Atenolol[3] – generic[4]	25, 50, 100 mg tabs	25-100 mg in
Tenormin (AstraZeneca)		1 or 2 doses
Betaxolol[3] – generic	10, 20 mg tabs	5-40 mg once
Bisoprolol[3] – generic	5, 10 mg tabs	5-20 mg once
Zebeta (Teva)		
Metoprolol[3] – generic[4]	25, 50, 100 mg tabs	50-200 mg in
Lopressor (Novartis)		1 or 2 doses
extended-release	50, 100 mg tabs	
Toprol-XL (AstraZeneca)	25, 50, 100, 200 mg ER tabs	25-400 mg once
Nadolol – generic[4]	20, 40, 80 mg tabs	20-320 mg once
Corgard (Pfizer)		
Propranolol – generic[4]	10, 20, 40, 60, 80 mg tabs	40-240 mg in
Inderal (Akrimax)		2 doses
extended-release	60, 80, 120, 160 mg ER caps	60-240 mg once
generic		
Inderal LA (Akrimax)		
InnoPran XL (GSK)	80, 120 mg ER caps	80-120 mg at
		bedtime
Timolol – generic	5, 10, 20 mg tabs	10-60 mg in
		2 doses
BETA BLOCKERS WITH INTRINSIC SYMPATHOMIMETIC ACTIVITY		
Acebutolol[3] – generic	200, 400 mg caps	200-1200 mg in
Sectral (Dr. Reddy's Labs)		1 or 2 doses
Penbutolol – *Levatol*	20 mg tabs	10-80 mg once
(UCB Pharma)		
Pindolol – generic	5, 10 mg tabs	10-60 mg in
		2 doses

1. FDA pregnancy categories: A = controlled studies show no risk; B = no evidence of risk; C = risk cannot be ruled out; D = positive evidence of risk; X = contraindicated in pregnancy
2. In addition to the adverse effects listed, antihypertensive drugs may interact adversely with other drugs.

Pregnancy Category[1]	Frequent or Severe Adverse Effects[2]
D	
C	
C	
C	Fatigue, depression, bradycardia, erectile dysfunction, decreased exercise tolerance, heart failure, worsening of peripheral arterial insufficiency, may aggravate allergic reactions, bronchospasm, may mask symptoms of and delay recovery from hypoglycemia,
C	Raynaud's phenomenon, insomnia, vivid dreams or hallucinations, acute mental disorder, increased serum triglycerides,
C	decreased HDL cholesterol, increased incidence of diabetes, sudden withdrawal may lead to exacerbation of angina and myocardial infarction
C	
B	
C	Similar to other beta-adrenergic blocking drugs, but with less resting bradycardia and lipid changes, acebutolol has been associated with a positive antinuclear antibody test and occa-
B	sional drug-induced lupus

3. Cardioselective
4. A 30-day supply of some strengths is available for $4 at some discount pharmacies.

Continued on next page.

Drugs for Hypertension

BETA-ADRENERGIC BLOCKERS (continued)

Drug	Some Oral Formulations	Usual Daily Maintenance Dosage
BETA BLOCKERS WITH ALPHA-BLOCKING ACTIVITY		
Carvedilol – generic[4]	3.125, 6.25, 12.5, 25 mg tabs	12.5-50 mg in
Coreg (GSK)		2 doses
extended-release		
Coreg CR (GSK)	10, 20, 40, 80 mg ER tabs	20-80 mg once
Labetalol – generic	100, 200, 300 mg tabs	200-1200 mg in
		2 doses
Trandate (Prometheus)	100, 200 mg tabs	
BETA BLOCKERS WITH VASODILATING NITRIC-OXIDE-MEDIATED ACTIVITY		
Nebivolol – *Bystolic*	2.5, 5, 10, 20 mg tabs	5-40 mg once
(Forest)		

DIRECT VASODILATORS

Direct vasodilators frequently produce reflex tachycardia and rarely cause orthostatic hypotension. They should usually be given with a beta blocker or a centrally-acting drug to minimize the reflex increase in heart rate and cardiac output, and with a diuretic to avoid sodium and water retention. They should generally be avoided in patients with coronary artery disease. **Hydralazine** maintenance dosage should be limited to 200 mg per day to decrease the possibility of a lupus-like reaction. **Minoxidil**, a potent drug that rarely fails to lower blood pressure, should be reserved for severe hypertension refractory to other drugs. It causes hirsutism and tachycardia and can also cause severe fluid retention.

Pregnancy Category[1]	Frequent or Severe Adverse Effects[2]
C	
C	Similar to other beta-adrenergic blocking drugs, but more orthostatic hypotension; hepatotoxicity
C	Similar to other beta-adrenergic blocking drugs but may not cause impotence and may improve erectile dysfunction.

PERIPHERAL ADRENERGIC NEURON ANTAGONISTS

Reserpine is an effective antihypertensive but is seldom used now because (in doses much higher than currently recommended) it can cause severe depression.[35] **Guanadrel** (no longer available in the US) decreases cardiac output and may lower systolic pressure more than diastolic; postural and exertional hypotension occur commonly and are aggravated by vasodilatation caused by heat, exercise or alcohol.

COMBINATION THERAPY

Most patients with hypertension eventually need more than one drug to control their BP. Patients with a BP >20/10 mm Hg at baseline may bene-

Continued on page 163

ALPHA-ADRENERGIC BLOCKERS AND OTHER ANTIHYPERTENSIVES

Drug	Some Formulations	Usual Daily Maintenance Dosage
ALPHA-ADRENERGIC BLOCKERS		
Doxazosin – generic[3]	1, 2, 4, 8 mg tabs	1-16 mg once[4]
Cardura (Pfizer)		
Prazosin – generic[3]	1, 2, 5 mg caps	1-20 mg in
Minipress (Pfizer)		2 or 3 doses[4]
Terazosin – generic[3]	1, 2, 5, 10 mg caps	1-20 mg once[4]
Hytrin (Abbott)		
CENTRAL ALPHA-ADRENERGIC AGONISTS		
Clonidine – generic[3]	0.1, 0.2, 0.3 mg tabs	0.1-0.6 mg in
Catapres		2 or 3 doses
(Boehringer Ingelheim)		
transdermal – generic	0.1, 0.2, 0.3 mg patches	one patch weekly
Catapres TTS (transdermal)		(0.1 to 0.3 mg/day)
Guanfacine – generic[3]	1, 2 mg tabs	1-3 mg once
Methyldopa – generic[3]	250, 500 mg tabs	250 mg-2 g in 2 doses
DIRECT VASODILATORS		
Hydralazine – generic[3]	10, 25, 50, 100 mg tabs	40-200 mg in 2-4 doses
Minoxidil – generic	2.5, 10 mg tabs	2.5-40 mg in
		1 or 2 doses
PERIPHERAL ADRENERGIC NEURON ANTAGONISTS		
Reserpine – generic	0.1, 0.25 mg tabs	0.05-0.1 mg once

1. FDA pregnancy categories: A = controlled studies show no risk; B = no evidence of risk; C = risk cannot be ruled out; D = positive evidence of risk; X = contraindicated in pregnancy
2. In addition to the adverse effects listed, antihypertensive drugs may interact adversely with other drugs.

Pregnancy Category[1]	Frequent or Severe Adverse Effects[2]
C	
C	Syncope with first dose (less likely with terazosin and doxazosin), dizziness and vertigo, headache, palpitations, fluid retention, drowsiness, weakness, anticholinergic effects, priapism, thrombocytopenia, atrial fibrillation
C	
C	CNS reactions similar to methyldopa, but more sedation and dry mouth; bradycardia, heart block, rebound hypertension (less likely with patch), contact dermatitis from patch
B	Similar to clonidine, but milder
B	Sedation, fatigue, depression, dry mouth, orthostatic hypotension, bradycardia, heart block, autoimmune disorders (including colitis, hepatitis), hepatic necrosis, Coombs-positive hemolytic anemia, lupus-like syndrome, thrombocytopenia, red cell aplasia, impotence
C	Tachycardia, aggravation of angina, headache, dizziness, fluid retention, nasal congestion, lupus-like syndrome, hepatitis
C	Tachycardia, aggravation of angina, marked fluid retention, pericardial effusion, hair growth on face and body
C	Nasal stuffiness, drowsiness, GI disturbances, bradycardia, depression, nightmares with high doses, tardive dyskinesia

3. A 30-day supply of some strengths is available for $4 at some discount pharmacies.
4. The first dose is 1 mg at bedtime.

Drugs for Hypertension

SOME COMBINATION PRODUCTS

Drug	Strengths (mg)
ACE INHIBITORS AND DIURETICS	
Benazepril/HCTZ	5/6.25, 10/12.5, 20/12.5, 20/25 tabs
generic	
Lotensin HCT (Novartis)	
Captopril/HCTZ	25/15, 25/25, 50/15, 50/25 tabs
generic	
Capozide (Apothecon)	
Enalapril/HCTZ	5/12.5, 10/25 tabs
generic[1]	
Vaseretic (Biovail)	
Fosinopril/HCTZ	10/12.5, 20/12.5 tabs
generic	
Lisinopril/HCTZ	10/12.5, 20/12.5, 20/25 tabs
generic[1]	
Prinzide[2] (Merck)	
Zestoretic (AstraZeneca)	
Moexipril/HCTZ	7.5/12.5, 15/12.5, 15/25 tabs
generic	
Uniretic (UCB)	
Quinapril/HCTZ	10/12.5, 20/12.5, 20/25 tabs
generic	
Accuretic (Pfizer)	
ANGIOTENSIN RECEPTOR BLOCKERS AND DIURETICS	
Azilsartan/chlorthalidone	40/12.5, 40/25 tabs
Edarbyclor (Takeda)	
Candesartan/HCTZ	16/12.5, 32/12.5, 32/25 tabs
Atacand HCT (AstraZeneca)	
Eprosartan/HCTZ	600/12.5, 600/25 tabs
Teveten HCT (Abbott)	
Irbesartan/HCTZ	150/12.5, 300/12.5 tabs
Avalide (BMS)	
Losartan/HCTZ	50/12.5, 100/12.5, 100/25 tabs
Hyzaar (Merck)	

1. A 30-day supply of some strengths is available for $4 at some discount pharmacies.
2. Only available in 10/12.5 and 20/12.5 mg tabs

Drug	Strengths (mg)
ANGIOTENSIN RECEPTOR BLOCKERS AND DIURETICS (continued)	
Olmesartan/HCTZ	20/12.5, 40/12.5, 40/25 tabs
Benicar HCT (Daiichi Sankyo)	
Telmisartan/HCTZ	40/12.5, 80/12.5, 80/25 tabs
Micardis HCT (Boehringer Ingelheim)	
Valsartan/HCTZ	80/12.5, 160/12.5, 160/25, 320/12.5,
Diovan HCT (Novartis)	320/25 tabs
ARB AND DIRECT RENIN INHIBITOR	
Valsartan/aliskiren	160/150, 320/300 tabs
Valturna (Novartis)	
DIRECT RENIN INHIBITOR AND DIURETIC	
Aliskiren/HCTZ	150/12.5, 150/25, 300/12.5, 300/25 tabs
Tekturna HCT (Novartis)	
BETA-ADRENERGIC BLOCKERS AND DIURETICS	
Atenolol/chlorthalidone	50/25, 100/25 tabs
generic[1]	
Tenoretic (AstraZeneca)	
Bisoprolol/HCTZ	2.5/6.25, 5/6.25, 10/6.25 tabs
generic[1]	
Ziac (Duramed)	
Metoprolol/HCTZ	
generic	25/50, 25/100, 50/100 tabs
Lopressor HCT (Novartis)	25/50, 25/100 tabs
Nadolol/bendroflumethiazide	40/5, 80/5 tabs
generic	
Corzide (King)	
CALCIUM CHANNEL BLOCKERS AND ACE INHIBITORS	
Amlodipine/benazepril	2.5/10, 5/10, 5/20, 5/40, 10/20,
Lotrel (Novartis)	10/40 caps
Verapamil ER/trandolapril	180/2, 240/1, 240/2, 240/4 tabs
Tarka (Abbott)	

Continued on next page.

Drugs for Hypertension

SOME COMBINATION PRODUCTS (continued)

CALCIUM CHANNEL BLOCKERS AND ARBs	
Amlodipine/telmisartan –	5/40, 5/80, 10/40, 10/80 tabs
Twynsta (Boehringer Ingelheim)	
Drug	**Strengths (mg)**
CALCIUM CHANNEL BLOCKERS AND ARBs (continued)	
Amlodipine/valsartan	5/160, 5/320, 10/160, 10/320 tabs
Exforge (Novartis)	
Amlodipine/olmesartan	5/20, 5/40, 10/20, 5/40 tabs
Azor (Daiichi Sankyo)	
CALCIUM CHANNEL BLOCKERS AND DIRECT RENIN INHIBITOR	
Amplodipine/aliskiren	5/150, 10/150, 5/300, 10/300 tabs
Tekamlo (Novartis)	
DIURETIC COMBINATIONS	
HCTZ/spironolactone	
generic	25/25 tabs
Aldactazide (Pfizer)	25/25, 50/50 tabs
HCTZ/triamterene	
generic[1]	25/37.5, 25/50, 50/75 tabs, caps
Dyazide (GSK)	25/37.5 caps
Maxzide (Mylan)	25/37.5, 50/75 tabs
HCTZ/amiloride	50/5 tabs
generic[1]	
DIRECT VASODILATOR AND DIURETIC	
Hydralazine/HCTZ	25/25, 50/50 caps
Hydra-Zide (Par)	
CENTRAL ALPHA ADRENERGIC AGONIST AND DIURETIC	
Clonidine/chlorthalidone	0.1/15, 0.2/15, 0.3/15 tabs
Clorpres (Mylan)	
TRIPLE DRUG COMBINATIONS	
Aliskiren/amlodipine/HCTZ	150/5/12.5, 300/5/12.5, 300/5/25,
Amturnide (Novartis)	300/10/12.5, 300/10/25 tabs
Valsartan/amlodipine/HCTZ	160/5/12.5, 160/5/25, 160/10/12.5,
Exforge HCT (Novartis)	160/10/25, 320/10/25 tabs
Olmesartan/amlodipine/HCTZ	20/5/12.5, 40/5/12.5, 40/5/25, 40/10/12.5,
Tribenzor (Daiichi Sankyo)	40/10/25 tabs

fit from initiating therapy with 2 drugs.[36] By combining drugs with different mechanisms of action, lower doses can be used to effectively reduce BP and decrease the incidence of adverse effects.[37] Fixed-dose combination products (see Table) are widely available and may improve adherence. Three triple combination products are now available containing hydrochlorothiazide (12.5-25 mg) and amlodipine added to either aliskiren, olmesartan or valsartan.[38,39]

COST

Many of the drugs commonly used to treat hypertension are available generically. Some of these are available in large discount pharmacies for $4-10 for a 30-day supply.

1. Clevidipine (Cleviprex) for IV treatment of severe hypertension. Med Lett Drugs Ther 2008; 50:73.
2. Cardiovascular drugs in the ICU. Treat Guidel Med Lett 2002; 1:19.
3. BL Carter et al. Hydrochlorothiazide versus chlorthalidone: evidence supporting their interchangeability. Hypertension 2004; 43:4.
4. ME Ernst and M Moser. Use of diuretics in patients with hypertension. N Engl J Med 2009; 361:2153.
5. FH Messerli and S Bangalore. Half a century of hydrochlorothiazide: facts, fads, fiction and follies. Am J Med 2011; 124:896.
6. ALLHAT Officers and Coordinators for the ALLHAT Collaborative Research Group. Major outcomes in high-risk hypertensive patients randomized to angiotensin-converting enzyme inhibitor or calcium channel blocker vs diuretic: The Antihypertensive and Lipid-Lowering Treatment to Prevent Heart Attack Trial (ALLHAT). JAMA 2002; 288:2981.
7. JT Wright Jr et al. ALLHAT Collaborative Research Group. ALLHAT findings revisited in the context of subsequent analyses, other trials, and meta-analyses. Arch Intern Med 2009; 169:832.
8. Edarbyclor: an ARB/chlorthalidone combination for hypertension. Med Lett Drugs Ther 2012; 54:17.
9. NS Beckett et al. Treatment of hypertension in patients 80 years of age or older. N Engl J Med 2008; 358:1887.
10. DA Calhoun et al. Resistant hypertension: diagnosis, evaluation, and treatment: a scientific statement from the American Heart Association Professional Education Committee of the Council for High Blood Pressure Research. Circulation 2008; 117:e510.
11. Eplerenone (Inspra). Med Lett Drugs Ther 2003; 45:39.
12. GS Francis and WH Tang. Should we consider aldosterone as the primary screening target for preventing cardiovascular events? J Am Coll Cardiol 2005; 45:1249.

Drugs for Hypertension

13. Drugs for treatment of chronic heart failure. Treat Guidel Med Lett 2009; 7:53.
14. R Kunz et al. Meta-analysis: effect of monotherapy and combination therapy with inhibitors of the renin angiotensin system on proteinuria in renal disease. Ann Intern Med 2008; 148:30.
15. LM Wing et al. A comparison of outcomes with angiotensin-converting--enzyme inhibitors and diuretics for hypertension in the elderly. N Engl J Med 2003; 348:583.
16. HH Parving et al. The effect of irbesartan on the development of diabetic nephropathy in patients with type 2 diabetes. N Engl J Med 2001; 345:870.
17. EJ Lewis et al. Renoprotective effect of the angiotensin-receptor antagonist irbesartan in patients with nephropathy due to type 2 diabetes. N Engl J Med 2001; 345:851.
18. BM Brenner et al [RENAAL]. Effects of losartan on renal and cardiovascular outcomes in patients with type 2 diabetes and nephropathy. N Engl J Med 2001; 345:861.
19. B Dahlöf et al. Cardiovascular morbidity and mortality in the Losartan Intervention For Endpoint reduction in hypertension study (LIFE): a randomised trial against atenolol. Lancet 2002; 359:995.
20. JN Cohn, G Tognoni, Valsartan Heart Failure Trial Investigators. A randomized trial of the angiotensin-receptor blocker valsartan in chronic heart failure. N Engl J Med 2001; 345:1667.
21. MA Pfeffer et al. Valsartan, captopril, or both in myocardial infarction complicated by heart failure, left ventricular dysfunction, or both. N Engl J Med 2003; 349:1893.
22. JB Young et al. Mortality and morbidity reduction with candesartan in patients with chronic heart failure and left ventricular systolic dysfunction: results of the CHARM low-left ventricular ejection fraction trials. Circulation 2004; 110:2618.
23. S Yusuf et al. Telmisartan, ramipril, or both in patients at high risk for vascular events. N Engl J Med 2008; 358:1547.
24. Aliskiren (Tekturna) for hypertension. Med Lett Drugs Ther 2007; 49:29.
25. S Oparil et al. Efficacy and safety of combined use of aliskiren and valsartan in patients with hypertension: a randomised, double-blind trial. Lancet 2007; 370:221.
26. Blood Pressure Lowering Treatment Trialists' Collaboration. Effects of different blood-pressure-lowering regimens on major cardiovascular events: results of prospectively-designed overviews of randomised trials. Lancet 2003; 362:1527.
27. S Julius et al. Outcomes in hypertensive patients at high cardiovascular risk treated with regimens based on valsartan or amlodipine: the VALUE randomised trial. Lancet 2004; 363:2022.
28. K Jamerson et al. Benazepril plus amlodipine or hydrochlorothiazide for hypertension in high-risk patients. N Engl J Med 2008; 359:2417.
29. CS Wiysonge et al. Beta-blockers for hypertension. Cochrane Database Syst Rev 2007; 24 (1):CD002003.
30. BM Psaty et al. Health outcomes associated with various antihypertensive therapies used as first-line agents: a network meta-analysis. JAMA 2003; 289:2534.
31. National Clinical Guideline Centre, National Institute for Health and Clinical Excellence. Hypertension: The clinical management of primary hypertension in adults: Clinical Guideline 127. www.nice.org.uk/nicemedia/live/13561/56007.pdf. Accessed December 16, 2011.

32. G Mancia et al. Reappraisal of European guidelines on hypertension management: a European Society of Hypertension Task Force document. J Hypertens 2009; 27:2121.
33. GL Bakris et al. Metabolic effects of carvedilol vs metoprolol in patients with type 2 diabetes mellitus and hypertension: a randomized controlled trial. JAMA 2004; 292:2227.
34. Nebivolol (Bystolic) for hypertension. Med Lett Drugs Ther 2008; 50:17.
35. HB Slim et al. Older blood pressure medications — do they still have a place? Am J Cardiol 2011; 108:316.
36. TA Kotchen. Expanding role for combination drug therapy in the initial treatment of hypertension? Hypertension 2011; 58:550.
37. DS Wald et al. Combination therapy versus monotherapy in reducing blood pressure: meta-analysis on 11,000 participants from 42 trials. Am J Med 2009; 122:290.
38. In brief: another three drug combination for hypertension. Med Lett Drugs Ther 2011; 53:28.
39. Tribenzor for hypertension. Med Lett Drugs Ther 2010; 52:70.
40. Aliskiren trial terminated. Med Lett Drugs Ther 2012; 54:5.

DRUGS FOR
Lipids

Original publication date – March 2011 (revised March 2012)

Drugs that lower low-density lipoprotein cholesterol (LDL-C) concentrations can prevent formation, slow progression and cause regression of atherosclerotic lesions. Lipid-regulating drugs must be taken indefinitely; when they are stopped, plasma lipoproteins return to pretreatment levels in 2-3 weeks.

STATINS — HMG-CoA reductase inhibitors (statins) inhibit the enzyme that catalyzes the rate-limiting step in cholesterol synthesis. The subsequent reduction in hepatic cholesterol leads to increased LDL receptor activity and increased clearance of LDL-C from the blood. Statins are more effective than other drugs in lowering LDL-C, and they also lower triglycerides. Most statins increase high-density lipoprotein cholesterol (HDL-C), but only modestly.

Statins also have other effects: they improve endothelial function, decrease platelet aggregation and reduce inflammation. Statins decrease serum concentrations of C-reactive protein (CRP), a marker for circulating inflammatory cytokines.

Clinical Studies — Primary Prevention – When taken by patients with risk factors (such as high LDL-C, low HDL-C, hypertension or diabetes) but no previous coronary heart disease, statins have been shown to reduce the risk of subsequent cardiovascular disease. A 10-year post-trial follow-up of primary prevention with pravastatin (WOSCOPS) showed a persistent reduction in coronary events in patients who had received pravastatin compared to those who had received placebo.[1] In another study (JUPITER), among 17,802 apparently healthy men and women with LDL-C <130 mg/dL (3.4 mmol/L), but CRP $\geq$2.0 mg/L, rosuvastatin significantly lowered the risk of myocardial infarction, stroke or cardiovascular death (hazard ratio 0.56) compared to placebo.[2]

Secondary Prevention – Controlled trials in patients with **coronary heart disease** have shown that recommended doses of statins can lower the incidence of cardiac events and stroke and decrease mortality from all causes, even in patients with normal LDL-C levels.[3] Among 4731 patients with a **recent stroke or TIA** and no coronary disease (SPARCL), atorvastatin 80 mg significantly decreased the number of recurrent strokes compared to placebo (265 vs. 311). The number of patients with ischemic stroke decreased by 56 while the number with hemorrhagic stroke increased by 22 with atorvastatin, both statistically significant changes.[4] Patients already on chronic statin therapy have shown evidence of beneficial cardioprotective effects from reloading, especially with high doses, at the time of percutaneous coronary intervention (PCI).[5,6] Perioperative statin therapy in patients undergoing vascular surgery has been associated with an improvement in postoperative cardiac outcomes.[7]

High- vs. Low-Dose – Among nearly 10,000 patients with **stable coronary disease** treated with 10 or 80 mg of atorvastatin daily for 5 years (TNT), the higher dose reduced LDL-C to 77 mg/dL (2.0 mmol/L), compared to 101 mg/dL (2.6 mmol/L) with the lower dose, and reduced major cardiovascular events by 22% (relative) and 2.2% (absolute). Total mortality was similar in both groups.[8] A second trial (IDEAL) included close to 9000 patients treated **after myocardial infarction** with 80 mg of atorvastatin or 20-40 mg of simvastatin for 5 years. Mean LDL-C fell to 81 mg/dL (2.1 mmol/L) with atorvastatin and 104 mg/dL (2.7 mmol/L) with simvastatin. Major coronary events (the primary endpoint) were insignificantly (p=0.07) reduced by atorvastatin 80 mg compared to the 2 simvastatin doses. Rates of all-cause, cardiovascular and non-cardiovascular deaths were similar in the 2 groups.[9]

Started within 10 days of hospitalization for **acute coronary syndrome**, atorvastatin 80 mg, compared to pravastatin 40 mg, for 18-36 months in 4162 patients (PROVE IT-TIMI 22) significantly reduced a composite of death, major cardiac events and stroke by 16% (relative) and 3.9% (absolute).[10] Started within 5 days after onset of acute coronary syndrome, a trial (A to Z) of simvastatin 40 mg/d for the first month followed by 80 mg/d thereafter, compared to placebo for the first 4 months followed by simvastatin 20 mg/d, failed to show that the higher dose produced a significant benefit in reducing the primary composite endpoint of cardiovascular death, myocardial infarction, readmission for acute coronary syndrome and stroke.[11]

LDL-C Targets – Two years of treatment with 40 mg of rosuvastatin (ASTEROID) reduced LDL-C by 53% to 61 mg/dL (1.6 mmol/L), increased HDL-C by 15% and led to significant regression of coronary atherosclerosis.[12] A meta-analysis of 4 large trials of patients with either stable or acute coronary disease showed that high-dose statin therapy, compared to standard doses, lowered LDL-C levels further and significantly reduced cardiovascular events.[13]

For high-risk patients, the National Cholesterol Education Program recommends that LDL-C be lowered to less than 100 mg/dL (2.6 mmol/L) or by at least 30-40%, but considers a value <70 mg/dL (1.8 mmol/L) an optional goal for patients at very high risk.

Adverse Effects – Statins are generally well tolerated. Some patients who cannot tolerate one statin may tolerate another. Mild gastrointestinal disturbances, headache or rash may occur. **Myopathy** ranging from myalgia to myositis, with or without increased serum creatine kinase (CK), is common. The risk of myopathy is closely related to the dose of the drug and even more closely to its concentration in serum.[14] Rarely, rhabdomyolysis and myoglobinemia leading to renal failure can occur. Whether the risk and severity of myopathy are uniformly dose-related with all statins is unclear.[15] In one randomized trial (SEARCH) in 6031 patients, the incidence of myopathy was 0.9% in patients taking 80 mg of simvastatin daily and 0.03% in those taking 20 mg of simvastatin daily.[16] A similar dose-relationship has not been reported with atorvastatin in clinical trials. CK values should be measured at baseline and subsequently if the patient develops myalgia; if levels exceed 3-5 times the upper limit of normal (ULN), some expert clinicians would lower the dose or discontinue the drug. Others would wait until CK levels reach 5-10 times ULN.

An **increase in plasma aminotransferase** activities to more than 3 times ULN occurs in 1-2% of patients taking higher doses of statins. Patients who develop biochemical hepatitis with one statin may be able to tolerate another or lower doses of the same one. Current recommendations for hepatic monitoring vary. One approach would be baseline evaluation of liver function and transaminase measurements after 3 months and annually thereafter, or more frequently if indicated. Statin treatment is safe in patients with moderately elevated transaminase values (up to 3 times the upper limit of normal) and can reduce cardiovascular morbidity and improve liver function.[17]

An observational study has suggested a rare association of statin use with polyneuropathy.[18] Other reports have described memory loss, sleep disturbances, impotence, gynecomastia, a lupus-like syndrome, acute and usually mild pancreatitis, insulin resistance and increased glycemia, but with all of these, the relationship between cause and effect is not clear.

A meta-analysis of 26 randomized controlled trials including at least 1000 patients each and a minimum median follow-up of 2-6 years found no increase in cancer incidence or deaths with statin therapy.[3]

Drug Interactions – Statin-induced myopathy is often caused by drug interactions. Simvastatin and lovastatin undergo extensive first-pass metabolism by CYP3A4 in the liver, and their plasma concentrations can be increased dramatically by concurrent use of strong CYP3A4 inhibitors such as itraconazole (*Sporanox*, and others), ketoconazole (*Nizoral*, and others), clarithromycin (*Biaxin*, and others), nefazodone, and many HIV protease inhibitors. According to recent label changes, simvastatin and lovastatin are now contraindicated for use with strong inhibitors of CYP3A4.[42,43] Grapefruit juice inhibits intestinal CYP3A4 and in large amounts (1 quart or more) may also increase plasma levels of simvastatin and lovastatin.

Atorvastatin undergoes less first-pass metabolism by CYP3A4 and most 3A4 inhibitors produce only small increases in its plasma concentration, but rhabdomyolysis has occurred. Fluvastatin is mainly metabolized by CYP2C9, and few interactions have been reported. Pravastatin and rosuvastatin are not metabolized by the cytochrome P450 system to a clinically significant extent and are least affected by other drugs.

Cyclosporine (*Sandimmune*, and others) taken concurrently increases serum concentrations of all statins and the risk of rhabdomyolysis, probably through inhibition of drug transporters such as OATP and P-glycoprotein. Gemfibrozil used concurrently inhibits metabolism of statins by interfering with statin glucuronidation, increasing the risk of rhabdomyolysis.

Choice of a Statin – Lovastatin, pravastatin and simvastatin are available generically. Atorvastatin is more potent and has a well-documented beneficial effect on clinical outcomes. Rosuvastatin may be even more effective than atorvastatin in lowering LDL-C, and the incidence of rhabdomyolysis with rosuvastatin to date has been similar to that with other statins, but less information is available on clinical outcomes. Pitavastatin has not been shown to offer any advantage in cholesterol-lowering over statins that are available generically and clinical outcome studies are lacking.[19]

FIBRIC ACID DERIVATIVES — Fibrates activate the nuclear transcription factor peroxisome proliferator activated receptor-alpha (PPAR-

Drugs for Lipids

STATINS

Drug	Formulations
Atorvastatin – *Lipitor* (Pfizer)	10, 20, 40, 80 mg tabs
Fluvastatin – *Lescol* (Novartis)	20, 40 mg capsules
extended-release – *Lescol XL*	80 mg tablet
Lovastatin – generic	10, 20, 40 mg tabs
Mevacor (Merck)	20, 40 mg tablets
extended release – *Altoprev* (Shionogi)	20, 40, 60 mg tabs
Pitavastatin – *Livalo* (Kowa)	1, 2, 4 mg tabs
Pravastatin – generic	10, 20, 40, 80 mg tabs
Pravachol (Bristol-Myers Squibb)	10, 20, 40, 80 mg tabs
Rosuvastatin – *Crestor* (AstraZeneca)	5, 10, 20, 40 mg tabs
Simvastatin – generic	5, 10, 20, 40, 80 mg tabs
Zocor (Merck)	5, 10, 20, 40, 80 mg tabs

1. For initial treatment of patients with only modest elevations of LDL-C or a history of poor tolerance for these drugs, some expert reviewers use lower doses. For patients who require a large reduction in LDL-C, some would use higher doses initially. Statins are generally most effective when taken in the evening.
2. Or 40 mg bid.
3. 10 mg initially for patients with renal or hepatic dysfunction.
4. Higher serum concentrations of rosuvastatin have been reported in Asian patients; an initial dose of 5 mg once daily is recommended.

FDA-Approved Usual Adult Daily Dosage[1]	Usual Decrease in LDL Cholesterol
Initial: 10-20 mg once	35–40%
Maximum: 80 mg once	50–60%
Initial: 20 mg once	20–25%
Maximum: 40 mg bid	30–35%
80 mg once	35–38%
Initial: 20 mg once	25–30%
Maximum: 80 mg once[2]	35–40%
Initial: 20 mg once	20–25%
Maximum: 60 mg once	40–45%
Initial: 2 mg once	35–40%
Maximum: 4 mg once	40–45%
Initial: 40 mg once[3]	30–35%
Maximum: 80 mg once	35–40%
Initial: 40 mg once[3]	30–35%
Maximum: 80 mg once	35–40%
Initial: 10-20 mg once[4,5]	45–50%
Maximum: 40 mg once[6]	50–60%
Initial: 20 mg once[7]	35–40%
Maximum: 80 mg once[8,9]	45–50%
Initial: 20 mg once[7]	35–40%
Maximum: 80 mg once[8,9]	45–50%

5. Patients with severe renal impairment not on hemodialysis should begin with 5 mg and not exceed 10 mg/day.
6. Not to exceed 20 mg/day in Asian patients (Clin Pharmacol 2005; 78:330).
7. Patients with severe renal impairment should start with 5 mg.
8. Only for patients taking 80 mg for ≥ 12 months without evidence of myopathy.
9. The maximum dose of simvastatin should be 10 mg daily in patients also taking amiodarone *(Cordarone)*, diltiazem *(Cardizem)* or verapamil *(Calan)* and 20 mg daily if taken with amlodipine *(Norvasc)* or ranolazine *(Ranexa)*.

alpha), which regulates genes that control lipid and glucose metabolism, inflammation, and endothelial function.[20] Gemfibrozil (*Lopid*, and others), fenofibrate (*Tricor*, and others), fenofibric acid *(Trilipix)* and bezafibrate (*Bezalip* – available in Canada, not in the US) lower triglycerides, usually by 25-50%, and may increase HDL-C. They may lower LDL-C, but when they decrease elevated triglycerides, LDL-C may increase. Patients for whom fibrates are particularly indicated include those with hypertriglyceridemia severe enough to be at risk for pancreatitis and those who have hypertriglyceridemia with low HDL-C.

Gemfibrozil – A 13-year post-trial follow-up of the 5-year Helsinki Heart Study showed that patients treated with gemfibrozil had a significant 23% reduction in coronary mortality.[21]

Fenofibrate – Taken once daily, fenofibrate may be more effective than gemfibrozil in lowering plasma LDL-C and triglycerides. A randomized trial (ACCORD) in 5518 patients with type 2 diabetes with a mean follow-up of 4.7 years found no significant differences in cardiovascular outcomes between use of simvastatin alone or in combination with fenofibrate.[22]

Bezafibrate – In a placebo-controlled trial in 3090 patients with stable angina or a previous myocardial infarction who had not been treated with statins, the incidence of myocardial infarction or sudden cardiac death after 6 years was 13.6% with bezafibrate versus 15% with placebo; this difference was not statistically significant.[23]

Fenofibric Acid – The active metabolite of fenofibrate, fenofibric acid is marketed separately as *Trilipix*. There is no evidence that it is more effective than any other fibric acid derivative in lowering triglyceride levels or increasing HDL-C. As with other fibrates, addition of fenofibric acid to a statin has not been shown to improve cardiovascular outcomes.[24]

Adverse Effects – Fibrates are generally well tolerated. Gastrointestinal problems are the most common complaint, mainly with gemfibrozil.

Cholelithiasis, hepatitis and (especially with gemfibrozil) myositis can occur.

Drug Interactions – Fibrates may potentiate the effect of oral anticoagulants and oral hypoglycemic agents. Gemfibrozil inhibits metabolism of most statins except fluvastatin and increases the risk of rhabdomyolysis. Fenofibrate does not inhibit statin metabolism and is much less likely to increase the risk of rhabdomyolysis. Fenofibrates are eliminated renally and should be used with caution in patients taking cyclosporine (*Neoral*, and others) and other drugs that could increase the risk of nephrotoxicity.

NIACIN (NICOTINIC ACID) — Niacin modifies all plasma lipoproteins and lipids favorably. It increases HDL-C by 15-35% and decreases triglycerides by 20-35%. It decreases total plasma and LDL-C 5-25%, changing small, dense LDL particles to large, buoyant forms.[25] It also decreases plasma levels of lipoprotein(a), another marker of cardiovascular risk.[26] One meta-analysis of 11 randomized controlled trials in a total of 6616 patients with hyperlipidemia found that niacin alone or in combination with a statin reduced carotid intima thickness and decreased the incidence of coronary events and stroke.[27]

Niacin is available in an immediate-release, quickly absorbed formulation, an extended-release preparation *(Niaspan)* absorbed over 8 hours, and a sustained-release formulation absorbed over 12-24 hours. Combinations of extended-release niacin with immediate-release lovastatin *(Advicor)* and simvastatin *(Simcor)* are available for use in patients with hyper-cholesterolemia or mixed dyslipidemia.[28]

Adverse Effects – Niacin can cause skin flushing and pruritus, gastrointestinal distress, blurred vision, fatigue, glucose intolerance, hyperuricemia, hepatic toxicity, exacerbation of peptic ulcer and, rarely, dry eyes or hyperpigmentation. Some adverse effects, particularly flushing, are more common with the immediate-release formulation. Sustained-

Drugs for Lipids

NON-STATINS

Drug	Formulations
BILE ACID SEQUESTRANTS	
Colesevelam – *Welchol* tablets (Daiichi Sankyo)	625 mg tabs
Welchol packets	1.875 g/packet, 3.75 g/packet
Colestipol – generic	1 g tabs
Colestid tablets (Pfizer)	
Colestid packets	5 g/packet
Cholestyramine – generic (packets)	4 g/packet
Questran (Par)	
generic light (packets)	
Questran Light	
generic (granules)	4 g/dose
Questran	
CHOLESTEROL ABSORPTION INHIBITOR	
Ezetimibe – *Zetia* (Merck/Schering-Plough)	10 mg tabs
FIBRATES	
Gemfibrozil – generic	600 mg tabs
Lopid (Pfizer)	
Fenofibrate[1] – non-micronized	
generic	54, 160 mg tabs
Fenoglide (Sciele)	40, 120 mg tabs
Lipofen (Cipher)	50, 100, 150 mg caps
Lofibra (Gate)	54, 160 mg tabs
Tricor (Abbott)	48, 145 mg tabs
Triglide (Sciele)	50, 160 mg tabs
micronized – generic	67, 134, 200 mg caps
Antara (Oscient)	43, 130 mg caps
Lofibra (Gate)	67, 134, 200 mg caps
Fenofibric acid - *Trilipix* (Abbott)	45, 135 mg caps[2]
NIACIN	
Niacin immediate-release – OTC	500 mg tabs
extended-release – *Niaspan* (Abbott)	500, 750, 1000 mg ER tabs
sustained-release – *Slo-Niacin* (Upsher-Smith)	250, 500, 750 mg SR tabs

1. Generic fenofibrate products are also available. Micronized fenofibrate should be taken with food.
2. Delayed-release capsules.

Usual Adult Daily Dosage

3.75 g once or 1.875 g bid

10 g once or 5 g bid

8 g once or 4 g bid

10 mg once

600 mg bid

160 mg once
120 mg once
150 mg once
160 mg once
145 mg once
160 mg once
200 mg once
130 mg once
200 mg once
135 mg once

1000 mg tid
1000 mg once[3]
1000 mg bid

3. Taken with a low-fat snack at bedtime.

Continued on next page.

Drugs for Lipids

NON-STATINS (continued)

Drug	Formulations
FISH OIL CAPSULES	
Lovaza (GSK)	caps[4]
USP-verified fish oil capsules[6]	caps[7]

4. Each 1 gram capsule contains 465 mg EPA, 375 mg DHA (total 900 mg polyunsaturated fatty acids [PUFAs]).
5. FDA-approved dose for treating hypertriglyceridemia (≥500 mg/dL).
6. USP-verified fish oil products are manufactured by Berkley & Jensen, Equaline, Kirkland, Nature Made and NutriPlus.

release preparations have been hepatotoxic in doses of ≥ 2 grams per day. Flushing has been less frequent and hepatotoxicity has seldom been reported with the extended-release preparation in daily doses up to 2 grams. The cutaneous reactions can be diminished by starting with a low dose, taking niacin after meals, and taking aspirin (325 mg) or ibuprofen (200 mg) first.

CHOLESTEROL ABSORPTION INHIBITOR — Ezetimibe (*Zetia* in US; *Ezetrol* in Canada) inhibits intestinal absorption of both dietary and biliary cholesterol by blocking its transport at the brush border of the small intestine.[29] The recommended dose of 10 mg/day reduces LDL-C by about 18%. A fixed-dose combination of ezetimibe and simvastatin (*Vytorin*)[30] lowers LDL-C by 20-65%, depending on the simvastatin dose. A 2-year study (ENHANCE) in 720 patients with heterozygous familial hypercholesterolemia (mean baseline LDL-C 318 mg/dL) comparing ezetimibe 10 mg plus simvastatin 80 mg with simvastatin 80 mg alone found no significant difference in the primary endpoint of change in carotid intima-media thickness. LDL-C decreased significantly more with ezetimibe (58% vs. 41%).[31] No published data are available to date showing that ezetimibe alone or in combination with a statin improves cardiovascular outcomes.

178

Usual Adult Daily Dosage

4 caps once or 2 caps bid[5]
4 caps tid

7. Each 1 g capsule contains 300 mg PUFAs (180 mg EPA and 120 mg DHA); Nature Made Capsules are 1.2 g containing 360 mg PUFAs (216 mg EPA and 144 mg DHA). Three capsules are approximately equal to one *Lovaza* capsule.

Adverse Effects – Ezetimibe has generally been well tolerated. Severe diarrhea has been reported. Myalgia, rhabdomyolysis, severe hepatitis, pancreatitis and thrombocytopenia have also been reported.[32,33] According to the package insert, patients with moderate to severe hepatic insufficiency may have increased serum concentrations of the drug and should not take it.

Drug Interactions – Ezetimibe may increase the anticoagulant effect of warfarin. Bile acid sequestrants interfere with absorption of ezetimibe and, if used concurrently, they should be taken at least several hours apart. Cyclosporine increases plasma levels of ezetimibe; the clinical significance is unknown.

BILE ACID SEQUESTRANTS — The resins cholestyramine (*Questran*, and others) and colestipol (*Colestid*, and others) and the hydrophilic polymer colesevelam hydrochloride *(Welchol)*[34] are not absorbed from the gastrointestinal tract. These drugs can lower LDL-C by up to 20% and increase HDL-C, but may raise plasma triglyceride concentrations in patients with hypertriglyceridemia. Cholestyramine has been shown to reduce the number of cardiovascular events, but no clinical outcome data are available for colestipol or colesevelam.

ADVERSE EFFECTS OF CHOLESTEROL-LOWERING DRUGS

STATINS
GI disturbances, headache, rash, fatigue, myalgia and muscle weakness leading to rhabdomyolysis, elevated hepatic enzymes, and hepatic dysfunction
Rare: Polyneuropathy, memory loss, sleep disturbances, impotence, gynecomastia, lupus-like syndrome, and pancreatitis

FIBRIC ACID DERIVATIVES
GI disturbances, cholelithiasis, hepatitis, and myositis

NIACIN
Skin flushing, pruritus, GI disturbances, blurred vision, fatigue, glucose intolerance, hyperuricemia, hepatic toxicity, and exacerbation of peptic ulcers (adverse effects, especially flushing, are more frequent with IR products)
Rare: Dry eyes and hyperpigmentation

EZETIMIBE
Abdominal pain, diarrhea, arthralgia, myalgia, rhabdomyolysis, hepatitis, pancreatitis, and thrombocytopenia

BILE ACID SEQUESTRANTS
Constipation, heartburn, nausea, eructation, and bloating (adverse effects are more common with colestipol and cholestyramine and may diminish over time)

Adverse Effects – The resins can decrease plasma folate levels, and supplementation should be considered in younger women and children. The adverse effects of colestipol and cholestyramine are similar; constipation occurs frequently and may be accompanied by heartburn, nausea, eructation and bloating. These symptoms may diminish over time. Increased dietary fiber or a fiber supplement (*Metamucil*, and others) may relieve constipation and bloating. Giving the drugs in moderate doses (8-10 g/d or less) just before meals improves tolerance, but decreases effectiveness.

Colesevelam is much better tolerated than cholestyramine or colestipol, with fewer gastrointestinal symptoms, and clinically meaningful decreased absorption of other drugs taken concurrently has not been reported to date.

Drug Interactions – A number of drugs, including statins, should be taken either 1-2 hours before or 4-6 hours after colestipol and cholestyramine.

FISH OIL — Long-chain, highly unsaturated omega-3 fatty acids, present in cold-water fish and commercially available in capsules, can decrease fasting triglyceride concentrations 20-50% by reducing hepatic triglyceride production and increasing triglyceride clearance.[35] With long-term intake, they may increase HDL-C. A large, randomized 5-year trial in 18,645 statin-treated, hypercholesterolemic Japanese patients showed a significant reduction in major coronary events (262 vs. 324) when 1.8 g of eicosapentanoic acid was added to statin therapy.[36] A trial in 4837 statin-treated patients who had previously had a myocardial infarction, found that addition of omega-3 fatty acids in margarine had no demonstrable cardioprotective effects.[37]

Lovaza – The first FDA-approved omega-3 product, *Lovaza* (formerly *Omacor*) is marketed in 1-g capsules and is approved for treatment of hypertriglyceridemia. In the recommended dosage of 4 g per day, it lowers triglycerides by 20-50%, but has not been shown to prevent pancreatitis. *Lovaza* is an alternative to fibrates for combination use with a statin. It does not increase the risk of rhabdomyolysis.

CHOLESTERYL ESTER TRANSFER PROTEIN INHIBITORS — A new class of drugs, cholesteryl ester transfer protein (CETP) inhibitors have been shown to dramatically reduce LDL cholesterol and increase HDL cholesterol. CETP is a plasma protein that promotes the transfer of cholesteryl esters from HDL and other lipoprotein fractions. The first CETP inhibitor that was studied, torcetrapib, caused cardiovascular events and death. The second, anacetrapib, reduced average LDL cholesterol from 81 mg/dL to 45 mg/dL, compared to 82 mg/dL to 77 mg/dL with placebo, in 1623 patients with, or at high risk for, coronary heart disease who were already taking a statin and, most remarkably, increased HDL cholesterol levels from 41 mg/dL to 101 mg/dL. Adverse effects seen with torcetrapib have not been reported with anacetrapib.[38] Dalcetrapib, another

Drugs for Lipids

CETP, raised HDL-C by 25-30% when used alone or in combination with a statin, with minimal effect on LDL-C.[39] The usefulness of these investigational agents for treatment of lipid disorders remains to be established. Whether the marked increase in HDL levels would have clinical benefits is unknown.

RED YEAST RICE — A fermented rice product that contains naturally occurring HMG-CoA reductase inhibitors is commercially available in capsules, but the amount of statin in each product can vary and, as with other dietary supplements, its production is not regulated by the FDA. In one study, the lipid-lowering effect of a red yeast rice product was equivalent to that of 20-40 mg of lovastatin.[40] Both myalgias and myopathy have been reported following use of red yeast rice.

COMBINATIONS — In high-risk patients with LDL-C treatment goals of <100 mg/dL (2.6 mmol/L), statin monotherapy is often not sufficient; addition of another LDL-C lowering drug such as ezetimibe or niacin may be necessary to achieve LDL-C goals.

Statins may be used in combination with fenofibrate, niacin, colesevelam or omega-3 fatty acids to lower triglycerides and increase HDL-C, in addition to lowering LDL-C. Although concurrent use of ezetimibe and a fibrate may normalize plasma lipids in patients with combined dyslipidemia, this combination might lead to gallbladder disease because both drugs increase biliary cholesterol excretion. In severe hypertriglyceridemia not adequately controlled by diet, fibrates and niacin may be used together, possibly in combination with omega-3 fatty acids. Since treatment of hypertriglyceridemia with a fibrate may increase LDL-C, it sometimes becomes necessary to add a statin to what was initially fibrate monotherapy.

PREGNANCY — Statins are contraindicated during pregnancy; congenital anomalies have been reported with lovastatin in some animal species and in a few human infants. Gemfibrozil and fenofibrate are ter-

STATIN COMBINATION PRODUCTS*

Drug	Strength
NIACIN ER/LOVASTATIN	
Advicor (Abbott)[1]	500/20 mg
	750/20 mg
	1000/20 mg
	1000/40 mg
NIACIN ER/SIMVASTATIN	
Simcor (Abbott)[2]	500/20 mg
	750/20 mg
	1000/20 mg
	500/40 mg
	1000/40 mg
EZETIMIBE/SIMVASTATIN	
Vytorin (Merck/Schering)[3]	10/10 mg
	10/20 mg
	10/40 mg
	10/80 mg

* In addition to the combinations listed in the table, some statins are also available in combination with drugs to treat other indications. Atorvastatin is available in combination with the calcium channel blocker amlodipine *(Caduet)*, and simvastatin is available with the antidiabetic drug sitagliptin *(Juvisync)*.
1. Usual daily dosage is 1-2 tablets. Maximum daily dosage is 2000/40 mg. Take with a low-fat snack at bedtime.
2. Usual daily dosage is 1000/20 mg to 2000/40 mg taken at bedtime.
3. Usual daily dosage is 1 tablet in the evening. Maximum daily ezetimibe dosage is 10 mg.

atogenic in animals. The safety of niacin in lipid-lowering doses is unknown. Cholestyramine and colestipol might interfere with absorption of important nutrients. Colesevelam appears to be safe in animal reproductive studies. Ezetimibe has caused skeletal defects in some animal studies. Niacin and *Lovaza* are classified as category C (risk cannot be ruled out) for use in pregnancy.

CONCLUSION — HMG-CoA reductase inhibitors (statins) are the lipid-regulating drugs of first choice for treatment of most patients with, or at risk for, coronary or other atherosclerotic vascular disease. They can decrease the incidence of major coronary events and death in such patients. Patients who have had cardiovascular events have been shown to benefit from high doses of statins that achieve ≥ 50% lowering of LDL-C. Patients with risk factors for cardiovascular disease may benefit from taking a statin even if they have normal LDL-C levels.

When choosing a statin, a major consideration should be the magnitude of LDL-C reduction required. If moderate lowering is needed, lovastatin, simvastatin, pravastatin or a low dose of atorvastatin (10 mg) would be a reasonable choice. Intense LDL-C reduction can be obtained by using atorvastatin or rosuvastatin. Atorvastatin 80 mg is the drug of choice for patients with acute coronary syndromes.

Additional LDL-C reductions can be achieved by combining statins with other LDL-C lowering drugs, such as colesevelam, niacin or ezetimibe, but clinical outcome studies of such combinations are lacking.[41] Colesevelam is tolerated much better than the resin bile acid sequestrants and does not interfere with intestinal absorption of other drugs.

For patients with combined dyslipidemia, combination of a statin with fenofibrate, niacin or fish oil is recommended. A reasonable choice of drugs for patients with low HDL-C and low LDL-C who are at risk for coronary disease would be niacin alone or in combination with a statin. Of the fibrate preparations available in the US, the clinical benefit is best documented for gemfibrozil, but gemfibrozil inhibits the metabolism of most statins, increasing the risk of rhabdomyolosis, while fenofibrate does not.

1. I Ford et al. Long-term follow-up of the West of Scotland Coronary Prevention Study. N Engl J Med 2007; 357:1477.
2. PM Ridker et al [JUPITER]. Rosuvastatin to prevent vascular events in men and women with elevated C-reactive protein. N Engl J Med 2008; 359: 2195.
3. Cholesterol Treatment Trialists' (CTT) Collaboration. Efficacy and safety of more intensive lowering of LDL cholesterol: a meta-analysis of data from 170,000 participants in 26 randomised trials. Lancet 2010; 376:1670.

4. P Amarenco et al. The Stroke Prevention by Aggressive Reduction in Cholesterol Levels [SPARCL] Investigators. High-dose atorvastatin after stroke or transient ischemic attack. N Engl J Med 2006; 355:549.
5. G Di Sciascio et al. Efficacy of atorvastatin reload in patients on chronic statin therapy undergoing percutaneous coronary intervention: results of the ARMYDA-RECAPTURE (Atorvastatin for Reduction of Myocardial Damage During Angioplasty) randomized trial. J Am Coll Cardiol 2009; 54:558.
6. Y Sun et al. Effect of different loading doses of atorvastatin on percutaneous coronary intervention for acute coronary syndromes. Can J Cardiol 2010; 26:481.
7. O Schouten et al. Fluvastatin and perioperative events in patients undergoing vascular surgery. N Engl J Med 2009; 361:980.
8. JC LaRosa et al [TNT]. Intensive lipid lowering with atorvastatin in patients with stable coronary disease. N Engl J Med 2005; 352:1425.
9. TR Pedersen et al [IDEAL]. High-dose atorvastatin vs usual-dose simvastatin for secondary prevention after myocardial infarction: the IDEAL study: a randomized controlled trial. JAMA 2005; 294:2437.
10. CP Cannon et al [PROVE IT-TIMI 22]. Intensive versus moderate lipid lowering with statins after acute coronary syndromes. N Engl J Med 2004; 350:1495.
11. JA de Lemos et al [A to Z Trial]. Early intensive vs a delayed conservative simvastatin strategy in patients with acute coronary syndromes: phase Z of the A to Z trial. JAMA 2004; 292:1307.
12. SE Nissen et al. [ASTEROID]. Effect of very high-intensity statin therapy on regression of coronary atherosclerosis: the ASTEROID trial. JAMA 2006; 295:1556.
13. CP Cannon et al. Meta-analysis of cardiovascular outcomes trials comparing intensive versus moderate statin therapy. J Am Coll Cardiol 2006; 48:438.
14. Drug interactions with simvastatin. Med Lett Drugs Ther 2008; 50:83.
15. MH Davidson and JG Robinson. Safety of aggressive lipid management. J Am Coll Cardiol 2007; 49:1753.
16. SEARCH Collaborative Group. Intensive lowering of LDL cholesterol with 80 mg versus 20 mg simvastatin daily in 12,064 survivors of myocardial infarction: a double-blind randomised trial. Lancet 2010; 376:1658.
17. VG Athyros et al. Safety and efficacy of long-term statin treatment for cardiovascular events in patients with coronary heart disease and abnormal liver tests in the Greek Atorvastatin and Coronary Heart Disease Evaluation (GREACE) Study: a post-hoc analysis. Lancet 2010; 376:1916.
18. D Gaist et al. Statins and risk of polyneuropathy: a case-control study. Neurology 2002; 58:1333.
19. Pitavastatin (Livalo) - the seventh statin. Med Lett Drugs Ther 2010; 52:57.
20. B Staels and JC Fruchart. Therapeutic roles of peroxisome proliferator-activated receptor agonists. Diabetes 2005; 54:2460.
21. L Tenkanen et al. Gemfibrozil in the treatment of dyslipidemia: an 18-year mortality follow-up of the Helsinki Heart Study. Arch Intern Med 2006; 166:743.
22. ACCORD Study Group. Effects of combination lipid therapy in type 2 diabetes mellitus. N Engl J Med 2010; 362:1563.

Drugs for Lipids

23. BIP Study Group. Secondary prevention by raising HDL cholesterol and reducing triglycerides in patients with coronary artery disease: the Bezafibrate Infarction Prevention (BIP) study. Circulation 2000; 102:21.
24. Fenofibric acid (Trilipix). Med Lett Drugs Ther 2009; 51:33.
25. JT Kuvin et al. Effects of extended-release niacin on lipoprotein particle size, distribution, and inflammatory markers in patients with coronary artery disease. Am J Cardiol 2006; 98:743.
26. BG Nordestgaard et al. Lipoprotein(a) as a cardiovascular risk factor: current status. Eur Heart J 2010; 31:2844.
27. E Bruckert et al. Meta-analysis of the effect of nicotinic acid alone or in combination on cardiovascular events and atherosclerosis. Atherosclerosis 2010; 201:363.
28. Simcor: A niacin/simvastatin combination. Med Lett Drugs Ther 2008; 50:25.
29. Three new drugs for hyperlipidemia. Med Lett Drugs Ther 2003; 45:17.
30. Vytorin: a combination of ezetimibe and simvastatin. Med Lett Drugs Ther 2004; 46:73.
31. JJ Kastelein et al. Simvastatin with and without ezetimibe in familial hypercholesterolemia. N Engl J Med 2008; 358:1431.
32. MF Stolk et al. Severe hepatic side effects of ezetimibe. Clin Gastroenterol Hepatol 2006; 4:908.
33. JM Havranek et al. Monotherapy with ezetimibe causing myopathy. Am J Med 2006; 119:285.
34. Colesevelam (Welchol) for hypercholesterolemia. Med Lett Drugs Ther 2000; 42:102.
35. Fish oil supplements. Med Lett Drugs Ther 2006; 48:59.
36. M Yokoyama et al. Effects of eicosapentaenoic acid on major coronary events in hypercholesterolaemic patients (JELIS): a randomized open-label, blinded endpoint analysis. Lancet 2007; 369:1090.
37. D Kromhout et al. N-3 fatty acids and cardiovascular events after myocardial infarction. N Engl J Med 2010; 363:2015.
38. CP Cannon et al. Safety of anacetrapib in patients with or at a high risk for coronary heart disease. N Engl J Med 2010; 363:2406.
39. JG Robinson. Dalcetrapib: a review of phase II data. Expert Opin Investig Drugs 2010; 19:795.
40. Red yeast rice. Med Lett Drugs Ther 2009; 51:71.
41. When a statin fails. Med Lett Drugs Ther 2009; 51:58.
42. New simvastatin dosing recommendations. Med Lett Drugs Ther 2011; 53:61.
43. Statin label changes. Med Lett Drugs Ther 2012; 54:21.

WHAT ABOUT NIACIN?

Originally published in The Medical Letter – November 2011; 53:93

The results of the AIM-HIGH trial conducted by the US National Heart, Lung and Blood Institute (NHLBI) were recently published.[1] The goal of the trial was to test whether addition of niacin to intensive statin therapy would further reduce the risk of cardiovascular disease. The trial was stopped prematurely after an average follow-up of 3 years because niacin therapy had not shown any clinical benefit.

NIACIN — Through several mechanisms of action, niacin favorably modifies all plasma lipoproteins and lipids.[2] It increases high-density lipoprotein cholesterol (HDL-C) by 15-35% and decreases triglycerides by 20-35%. It decreases total plasma and low-density lipoprotein cholesterol (LDL-C) by 5-25%, changing small, dense LDL particles to large, buoyant forms.[3]

THE AIM-HIGH TRIAL — A total of 3414 patients (85% men) with cardiovascular disease, low HDL-C and elevated triglycerides were randomized to receive extended-release niacin *(Niaspan)* 1500-2000 mg/day or placebo. All patients in both groups were given simvastatin *(Zocor)* 40-80 mg/day and, if needed, ezetimibe *(Zetia)* 10 mg/day to lower their LDL-C to the range of 40-80 mg/dL. The composite primary endpoint (death from coronary heart disease, nonfatal myocardial infarction, ischemic stroke, hospitalization for an acute coronary syndrome or symptom-driven coronary or cerebral revascularization) occurred in 282 patients (16.4%) taking niacin and in 274 (16.2%) taking placebo.[1]

AN OLDER CLINICAL TRIAL — The Coronary Drug Project conducted between 1966 and 1975 in men with a previous myocardial infarction (MI) and hypercholesterolemia found that niacin (n=1119) significantly reduced the incidence of non-fatal recurrent MI compared to placebo (n=2739), but did not decrease total mortality. Nine years after the end of the trial, however, the mortality among niacin-treated patients (a post-hoc secondary analysis of a non-primary endpoint) was 52.0% compared to 58.2% with placebo, a statistically significant difference.[4]

OTHER CLINICAL TRIALS — Combining the results of the Coronary Drug Project and 5 small clinical trials with cardiovascular endpoints using various combinations of niacin with other pharmacologic agents, niacin was significantly beneficial in all, except for one trial in patients with normal LDL-cholesterol levels (mean 138 mg/dL, considered normal at that time) at entry.[5] A meta-analysis of 11 randomized controlled trials (also including patients in the Coronary Drug Project) in a total of 6616 patients with hyperlipidemia found that niacin alone or in combination with a statin reduced carotid intima thickness and decreased the incidence of coronary events and stroke.[6]

ADVERSE EFFECTS — Niacin can cause skin flushing, pruritus, gastrointestinal distress, blurred vision, fatigue, glucose intolerance, hyperuricemia, hepatic toxicity, exacerbation of peptic ulcer and, rarely, dry eyes or hyperpigmentation. Flushing has been less frequent and hepatotoxicity has been rare with the extended-release preparation in daily doses up to 2 grams.

CONCLUSION — The results of the AIM-HIGH trial in patients with very low LDL cholesterol levels should not discourage practitioners from prescribing niacin for hypercholesterolemic patients at risk for cardiovascular disease.

1. The AIM-HIGH Investigators. Niacin in patients with low HDL cholesterol levels receiving intensive statin therapy. N Engl J Med. 2011 Nov 15 (epub).
2. VS Kamanna and ML Kashyap. Mechanism of action of niacin. Am J Cardiol 2008; 101:20B.
3. Drugs for lipids. Treat Guidel Med Lett 2011; 9:13.
4. PL Canner et al. Fifteen year mortality in Coronary Drug Project patients: long-term benefit with niacin. J Am Coll Cardiol 1986; 8:1245.
5. JR Guyton. Effect of niacin on atherosclerotic cardiovascular disease. Am J Cardiol 1998; 82:18U.
6. E Bruckert et al. Meta-analysis of the effect of nicotinic acid alone or in combination on cardiovascular events and atherosclerosis. Atherosclerosis 2010; 201:353.

DRUGS FOR
Pain

Original publication date – April 2010 (revised March 2012)

Pain can be acute or chronic. Chronic pain has been broadly classified into two types: nociceptive and neuropathic. Nociceptive pain can be treated with nonopioid analgesics or opioids. Neuropathic pain is less responsive to opioids; adjuvant medicines such as antidepressants and anticonvulsants are often used to treat neuropathic pain. Combining different types of analgesics may provide an additive analgesic effect without increasing adverse effects.

NONOPIOID ANALGESICS

The maximum analgesic effect of acetaminophen and aspirin usually occurs with single doses between 650 and 1300 mg. With nonsteroidal anti-inflammatory drugs (NSAIDs) other than aspirin, the analgesic ceiling may be higher. Tolerance does not develop to the analgesic effects of these drugs.

SALICYLATES — Aspirin is effective for most types of mild to moderate pain, but its principal use now is in low doses as a platelet inhibitor. Unlike other NSAIDs, a single dose of aspirin irreversibly inhibits platelet function for the 8- to 10-day life of the platelet, interfering with hemostasis and prolonging bleeding time. A single dose of aspirin can precipitate asthma in aspirin-sensitive patients. High doses or chronic use

Continued on page 194

Drugs for Pain

SOME NONOPIOID ANALGESICS FOR PAIN

Drug	Usual Analgesic Dose	Dose Interval
Acetaminophen[1] (*Tylenol*, others)	PO: 500-1000 mg	q4-6h
SALICYLATES Aspirin[1] (*Bayer*, others)	PO: 325-650 mg	q4-6h
Choline magnesium trisalicylate	PO: 750-1500 mg	q8-12h
Diflunisal (*Dolobid*, others)	PO: 1000 mg initial, then 500 mg	q8-12h
SOME NON-SELECTIVE NSAIDs Diclofenac potassium (*Cataflam*, others)	PO: 50 mg	q8h-12h
Zipsor	PO: 25 mg	q6h
Etodolac	PO: 200-400 mg	q6-8h
Flurbiprofen (*Ansaid*, others)	PO: 50-100 mg	q6-12h
Ibuprofen Rx	PO: 400 mg	q4-6h
Ibuprofen OTC[1] (*Advil*, others)	PO: 200-400 mg	q4-6h
Ibuprofen IV *(Caldolor)*	IV: 400-800 mg	q6h

1. Available without a prescription.

190

Maximum Daily Dose	Comments
4000 mg	1000 mg more effective than 650 mg in some patients. Also available as an IV formulation *(Ofirmev)*.
4000 mg	Available in chewable, buffered, enteric-coated and extended-release formulations.
3000 mg	Effectiveness compared to aspirin not clear; onset of analgesia probably slower; less gastropathy and no impairment of platelet function.
1500 mg	500 mg comparable to 650 mg of aspirin or acetaminophen with slower onset and longer duration.
150 mg	Comparable to aspirin with longer duration; available in enteric-coated and extended-release tabs (*Voltaren*, others);
100 mg	available with misoprostol *(Arthrotec)* to decrease GI toxicity; also approved as topical patch *(Flector)* for minor trauma; also approved as gel *(Voltaren 1% Gel)* for relief of pain of osteoarthritis in knees and hands.
1200 mg	200 mg comparable to ibuprofen 400 mg; possibly superior to 650 mg of aspirin; also available as extended relief.
300 mg	FDA-approved only for use in osteoarthritis and rheumatoid arthritis.
2400 mg	200 mg equal to 650 mg of aspirin or acetaminophen, 400 mg superior with longer duration; 400 mg comparable to acetaminophen/codeine combination; also available in combination with famotidine *(Duexis)*.
1200 mg	
3200 mg	Has a modest opioid-sparing effect. Effectiveness compared to ketorolac not clear.

Continued on next page.

SOME NONOPIOID ANALGESICS FOR PAIN (continued)

Drug	Usual Analgesic Dose	Dose Interval
SOME NON-SELECTIVE NSAIDs (continued)		
Ketoprofen[1]	PO: 25-50 mg	q6-8h
Ketorolac (*Toradol*, others)	IM or IV:	q6h
	Patients <65 yrs: 30 mg	q6h
	IM or IV:	
	Patients $\geq$65 yrs: 15 mg	
	PO: 10 mg	q4-6h
	Intranasal *(Sprix)*:	
	Patients <65 yrs: 1 spray (31.5 mg) in each nostril	q6-8h
	Patients $\geq$65 yrs: 1 spray (31.5 mg) in one nostril	q6-8h
Mefenamic acid (*Ponstel*)	PO: 500 mg initial, then 250 mg	q6h
Meloxicam (*Mobic*, others)	PO: 7.5-15 mg	q24h
Nabumetone	PO: 1000 mg initial, then 500-750 mg	q8-12h
Naproxen (*Naprosyn*, others)	PO: 500 mg initial, then 250 mg OR 500 mg	q6-8h q12h

Maximum Daily Dose	Comments
300 mg	25 mg comparable to ibuprofen 400 mg and superior to 650 mg of aspirin; 50 mg superior to acetaminophen/codeine combination. Also available as extended release by prescription.
120 mg 60 mg	Comparable to 12 mg IM morphine with longer duration; use should be limited to 5 days because of GI toxicity; can be given as a single IM dose of 60 mg (<65 yrs) or 30 mg ($\geq$65 yrs) or single IV dose of 30 mg (<65 yrs) and 15 mg ($\geq$ 65 yrs).
40 mg	10 mg comparable to aspirin or acetaminophen; 20 mg comparable to ibuprofen 400 mg; recommended only for continuation therapy after IM or IV ketorolac; total use not to exceed 5 days. Dose in patients weighing <50 kg or with renal impairment (GFR 30-90 mL/min) is 1 spray in one nostril. Maximum 4 doses/day for up to 5 days.
1250 mg	Comparable to aspirin, but more effective in dysmenorrhea; duration of use not to exceed 1 wk or 2-3 days for dysmenorrhea.
15 mg	FDA-approved only for use in osteoarthritis and rheumatoid arthritis.
2000 mg	FDA-approved only for use in osteoarthritis and rheumatoid arthritis.
1250 mg first day then 1000 mg	250 mg probably comparable to 650 mg of aspirin with longer duration; 500 mg superior to 650 mg of aspirin; also available as controlled release and enteric coated, and in a fixed-dose combination *(Vimovo)* with the proton pump inhibitor esomeprazole.

Continued on next page.

Drugs for Pain

SOME NONOPIOID ANALGESICS FOR PAIN (continued)

Drug	Usual Analgesic Dose	Dose Interval
SOME NON-SELECTIVE NSAIDs (continued)		
Naproxen sodium	PO: 550 mg initial then	
(*Anaprox*, others)	275 mg	q6-8h
	OR	
	550 mg	q12h
Naproxen sodium	PO: 220 or 440 mg initial, then	q8-12h
OTC[1] (*Aleve*, others)	220 mg	
SELECTIVE COX-2 INHIBITOR		
Celecoxib (*Celebrex*)	PO:400 mg initial, then	q24h
	200 mg	

of aspirin can cause gastropathy and salicylate intoxication. Aspirin should not be used during viral syndromes in children and teenagers because of the risk of Reye's syndrome.[1]

Nonacetylated salicylates such as choline magnesium trisalicylate do not interfere with platelet aggregation, are rarely associated with GI bleeding, and are well tolerated by asthmatic patients, but there are no controlled trials demonstrating their comparative efficacy for treatment of chronic pain.

ACETAMINOPHEN — Acetaminophen has no clinically significant anti-inflammatory activity and is less effective than full doses of NSAIDs, but also does not have their antiplatelet and adverse GI effects or their frequent renal and possible cardiovascular toxicity. Acetaminophen overdose can cause serious or fatal hepatic injury, and some patients, such as those who are fasting, concurrently taking isoniazid (INH), zidovudine (*Retrovir*, and others) or a barbiturate, or are heavy alcohol users, can develop hepatic

Maximum Daily Dose	Comments
1375 mg first day then 1100 mg	275 mg comparable to 650 mg of aspirin with longer duration; 550 mg superior to 650 mg of aspirin with longer duration. Also available as double-strength.
660 mg	440 mg comparable to 400 mg of ibuprofen with longer duration.
800 mg	Less effective than full doses of naproxen or ibuprofen.

injury after moderate overdosage or even high therapeutic doses. Most healthy patients can take up to 4 grams daily with no adverse effects, but in one study repeated use of such doses was associated with elevations in alanine aminotransferase (ALT) concentrations.[2] Acetaminophen may increase the anticoagulant effect of warfarin (*Coumadin*, and others).[3] In elderly patients, some clinicians have recommended lowering the maximum dosage of acetaminophen to 3 grams daily.[4]

Intravenous acetaminophen *(Ofirmev)* was recently approved by the FDA for management of pain either as monotherpapy (mild to moderate) or with an opioid (moderate to severe) and for reduction of fever.[51]

NON-SELECTIVE NSAIDs — NSAIDs inhibit cyclooxygenase (COX); non-selective NSAIDs inhibit both COX-1 and COX-2. In single full doses, most of the non-selective NSAIDs listed in the table on pages 190-195 are more effective analgesics than full doses of acetaminophen or aspirin for treatment of acute pain, and some have shown equal or greater analgesic effect than usual doses of an oral opioid combined with acetaminophen, or even injected opioids. Whether this is also true with repeated doses in chronic pain is less well established. Some patients may respond better to one NSAID than another.

Adverse Effects – The adverse effects of non-selective NSAIDs are qualitatively similar to those of aspirin. They can precipitate asthma and anaphylactoid reactions in aspirin-sensitive patients. Unlike aspirin, however, they cause reversible inhibition of platelet aggregation; platelet function returns when most of the drug has been eliminated. GI bleeding, ulceration and perforation can occur with all of these drugs, often without warning. High doses, prolonged use, previous peptic ulcer disease, excessive alcohol intake and advanced age increase the risk of these complications. A proton pump inhibitor such as omeprazole (*Prilosec*, and others) can reduce the risk of gastric ulcers in patients on chronic NSAID therapy.[5]

NSAIDs decrease synthesis of renal vasodilator prostaglandins and decrease renal blood flow, which can lead to fluid retention and may cause renal failure or hypertension; risk factors include advanced age, congestive heart failure, renal insufficiency, ascites, volume depletion and concurrent diuretic therapy. Hepatotoxicity can also occur.

Ibuprofen can interfere with the antiplatelet effect of aspirin. Patients taking aspirin for cardiovascular protection should not take ibuprofen regularly; single doses should be taken 2 hours after taking aspirin.

PARENTERAL NSAIDs — Ketorolac was the first NSAID to become available in an injectable formulation in the US; it is marketed for short-term (up to 5 days) analgesic use. Intramuscular or intravenous ketorolac is comparable in analgesic efficacy to moderate doses of morphine. Even with parenteral administration, severe GI toxicity such as bleeding, ulceration and perforation can occur, particularly in elderly patients.

Intravenous ibuprofen *(Caldolor)* was recently approved by the FDA for use in adults and is being marketed as an antipyretic and as an analgesic for moderate to severe pain, either alone or in conjunction with opioid therapy.[6]

SELECTIVE COX-2 INHIBITORS — Single-dose trials in patients with post-surgical dental pain have found 100-200 mg of celecoxib *(Celebrex)* more effective than placebo, but less effective than naproxen sodium 550 mg or ibuprofen 400 mg.[7]

Adverse Effects – Celecoxib appears to cause less GI toxicity than non-selective NSAIDs. Other adverse effects are similar to those of non-selective NSAIDs. Celecoxib does not inhibit platelet aggregation or increase bleeding time; if given with warfarin, it may increase INR and prothrombin time, but the effect is unlikely to be clinically significant.

OPIOIDS

Opioids can be divided into partial agonists, full agonists and mixed agonist/antagonists. The weaker full agonists—propoxyphene, hydrocodone, codeine and tramadol—are often prescribed in combination with nonopioid analgesics. Strong full agonists such as morphine, hydromorphone, oxymorphone, methadone, levorphanol, fentanyl and oxycodone are generally used for treatment of moderate to severe pain. Unlike NSAIDs, morphine and the other full agonists generally have no ceiling for their analgesic effectiveness except that imposed by adverse effects.

MORPHINE — Given orally, morphine is well absorbed but extensively metabolized on first pass through the liver, resulting in a low bioavailability of about 35%. Morphine should be used with caution in patients with

Drugs for Pain

severe renal insufficiency because accumulation of an active metabolite may cause agitation, confusion, delirium and other adverse effects.

Avinza, a long-acting oral formulation of morphine, combines immediate- and extended-release beads in capsules that can be opened for sprinkling on food such as applesauce; if the beads are crushed or chewed, a potentially fatal dose can be released. It is the only formulation of morphine that has a maximum daily limit (1600 mg) because of the renal toxicity of fumaric acid, one of the constituents of the beads. In a double-blind study, 30 mg of *Avinza* taken once daily was comparable to *MS Contin*, another long-acting formulation of morphine, 15 mg twice daily.[8]

A combination of morphine with naltrexone *(Embeda)* has been marketed with an indication for treatment of moderate to severe pain requiring around-the-clock analgesia; the addition of naltrexone is intended to prevent abuse of the opioid.[9]

OXYCODONE — Oxycodone, a semi-synthetic derivative of morphine, is only available in oral formulations. Oral oxycodone is about 9.5 times more potent than oral codeine and 1.5 times more potent than oral morphine.[10] For treatment of cancer pain, the long-acting formulation, *OxyContin*, has been equal in analgesic effect to the same total daily dose of short-acting oxycodone. Oxycodone has been similar in efficacy to morphine and hydromorphone for treatment of chronic pain due to cancer. No studies are available comparing multiple doses of oxycodone with other opioids such as methadone or fentanyl for treatment of chronic cancer pain.

OXYMORPHONE — A metabolite of oxycodone, oxymorphone was available in the US for many years only in parenteral and rectal formulations, but is now available in both short-acting *(Opana)* and long-acting *(Opana ER)* oral forms.[11] Long-acting oxymorphone provided adequate pain relief at a lower dose in cancer patients switched from long-acting morphine or oxycodone.[12] Patients taking long-acting oral oxymorphone should not consume alcohol because it can cause a substantial increase in the peak serum concentrations of the drug, which is 3 times more potent than oral morphine.

HYDROMORPHONE — A semi-synthetic opioid, hydromorphone (*Dilaudid*, and others) is available in parenteral, rectal and short- and long-acting oral formulations.

FENTANYL — Fentanyl (*Duragesic,*and others) is available for IV, intrathecal, epidural, transdermal and oral transmucosal use. **Transdermal** fentanyl offers a convenient delivery system for patients with chronic pain, particularly those with difficulty swallowing or malabsorption, but should be started only after initial titration with a short-acting opioid. Although usually re-applied every 72 hours, some patients need to change fentanyl patches every 48 hours to achieve adequate analgesia. As with other formulations of the drug, transdermal fentanyl can cause fatal respiratory depression. Patients should be warned that exposing the patch to heat, either from an external source, increased exertion, or possibly high fever could increase release of the drug.[13] Concomitant use of drugs that inhibit CYP3A4, especially strong inhibitors such as ketoconazole (*Nizoral*, and others) or clarithromycin (*Biaxin*, and others), can cause dangerous increases in serum concentrations of fentanyl.[14]

An **oral transmucosal** formulation *(Actiq)*, a fentanyl lozenge on a stick, is approved for treatment of breakthrough pain in cancer patients already taking strong opioids for persistent pain. Its absolute bioavailability is about 50%, divided equally between rapid absorption from the buccal mucosa and slower GI absorption. The appropriate dose is determined by starting with the lowest dose (200 mcg) and titrating upward; there is no apparent relationship between the total daily dose of opioids and the dose of transmucosal fentanyl required to manage breakthrough pain. Another transmucosal form of fentanyl for breakthrough pain is now available as an effervescent buccal tablet *(Fentora)*.[15] Doses of *Fentora* are lower than those of *Actiq* because of its increased bioavailability.[16,17] Fentanyl is also available in a buccal soluble film *(Onsolis),* a sublingual tablet

Continued on page 206

Drugs for Pain

SOME OPIOID ANALGESICS

Drug	Oral/Topical Formulations[1]
STRONG FULL AGONISTS	
Fentanyl	
Abstral (ProStrakan)	100, 200, 300, 400, 600, 800 mcg sublingual tabs
Actiq (Cephalon), others	0.2, 0.4, 0.6, 0.8, 1.2, 1.6 mg transmucosal lozenges
Duragesic (Janssen), others	12.5, 25, 50, 75, 100 mcg/hr transdermal patches
Fentora (Cephalon)	0.1, 0.2, 0.3, 0.4, 0.6, 0.8 mg buccal tabs
Lazanda (Archimedes)	100 mcg/100 mcL, 400 mcg/100 mcL nasal spray
Onsolis (Meda)	200, 400, 600, 800, 1200 mcg buccal films
Subsys (Insys)	100, 200, 400, 600, 800 mcg sublingual spray
Hydromorphone	
Dilaudid (Purdue), others	2, 4, 8 mg tabs; 5 mg/5 mL PO soln
Exalgo (Covidien)	8, 12, 16 mg ER tabs
Levorphanol	
Levo-Dromoran (Valeant), others	2 mg tabs
Meperidine	
Demerol (Sanofi aventis), others	50, 100 mg tabs; 50 mg/5mL syrup
Methadone	
Dolophine (Roxane), others	5, 10, mg tabs; 5, 10 mg/5 mL PO soln, 10 mg/mL PO conc; 40 mg dispersable tabs

1. See also "Some Opioid Combinations" table on page 209.

Duration of Action	Starting Oral Dose	Comments
≥ 1 hr ≥ 1 hr 72 hrs/patch ≥ 1 hr ≥ 1 hr ≥ 1 hr ≥ 1 hr	— — — — — — —	Not recommended for opioid-naive patients. Standard dose determined by previous opioid dosage. Also available parenterally (*Sublimaze*, and others). *Abstral, Actiq, Fentora* and *Onsolis* are indicated only for breakthrough pain. *Actiq* may cause dental caries.
4-6 hrs 24 hrs	2-8 mg —	Also available as a high potency injectable (*Dilaudid-HP*) and as a suppository.
6-8 hrs	2-4 mg	Accumulation may occur with chronic use.
3-4 hrs	50 mg	More rapid onset of action than morphine. Also available parenterally, but irritating to tissues. Toxic metabolite with long half-life causes CNS excitation and convulsions.
8-12 hrs	2.5-10 mg	Accumulation may occur with chronic use. Also available parenterally.

Continued on next page.

SOME OPIOID ANALGESICS (continued)

Drug	Oral/Topical Formulations[1]
STRONG FULL AGONISTS (continued)	
Morphine	15, 30 mg IR tabs
MS Contin (Purdue), others	15, 30, 60, 100, 200 mg ER tabs
Oramorph SR (Xanodyne)	15, 30, 60, 100 mg ER tabs
Kadian (Actavis)	10, 20, 30, 50, 60, 80, 100, 200 mg ER caps
Avinza (King)	30, 45, 60, 75, 90, 120 mg ER caps
Oxycodone	
Oxy IR (Purdue), others	5, 10, 15, 20, 30 mg IR tabs
Oxecta (King)	5, 7.5 mg tabs
OxyContin (Purdue)	10, 15, 20, 30, 40, 60, 80 mg ER tabs
Oxymorphone	
Opana (Endo)	5, 10 mg IR tabs
Opana ER	5, 7.5, 10, 15, 20, 30, 40 mg ER tabs
WEAK FULL AGONISTS	
Codeine	15, 30, 60 mg tabs
Hydrocodone	

Duration of Action	Starting Oral Dose	Comments
4-6 hrs	15-60 mg	Also available parenterally and as a suppository. Long-acting formulations not recommended for use in opioid-naive patients. Starting dose determined by previous opioid dosage. To avoid excessive release of the drug, *Avinza* and *Kadian* should not be taken with alcohol.
8-12 hrs	15-30 mg	
8-12 hrs	15-30 mg	
12 hrs	—	
24 hrs	—	
4-6 hrs	5-10 mg	
4-6 hrs	5-15 mg	
12 hrs	—	Long-acting formulations not recommended for opioid-naive patients. Starting dose determined by previous opioid dosage. ER formulations – biphasic absorption; 38% rapid, 62% slow.
		Also available parenterally.
4-6 hrs	5-20 mg	
12 hrs	5 mg	Long-acting formulations not recommended for opioid-naive patients. Starting dose determined by previous opioid dosage. No CYP50 drug interactions.
4 hrs	15-60 mg	60 mg PO equivalent to 650 mg of aspirin or acetaminophen; 10% of people lack the enzyme needed to make codeine active.
4 hrs	5-10 mg	10 mg PO equivalent to codeine 60-80 mg PO; only available in combinations.

Continued on next page.

SOME OPIOID ANALGESICS (continued)

Drug	Oral/Topical Formulations[1]
WEAK FULL AGONISTS (continued)	
Propoxyphene HCl[4]	
Darvon (Xanodyne), others	65 mg caps
Propoxyphene napsylate[4]	
Darvon-N (Xanodyne)	100 mg tabs
WEAK AGONIST/REUPTAKE INHIBITOR	
Tramadol	
Ultram (Ortho-McNeil Janssen), others	50 mg IR tabs
Ultram ER (Ortho-McNeil Janssen)	100, 200, 300 mg ER tabs
Ryzolt (Purdue)	
Tapentadol	
Nucynta (Ortho-McNeil Janssen)	50, 75, 100 mg tabs

2. Not to exceed 390 mg/day.
3. Not to exceed 600 mg/day.
4. Products containing propoxyphene are no longer available in the US.

Duration of Action	Starting Oral Dose	Comments
4 hrs	65 mg[2]	65 mg PO equivalent to codeine 32 mg PO; accumulation of metabolites can lead to CNS, cardiac and respiratory depression. Convulsions, cardiotoxicity and fatal overdose have occurred.
4 hrs	100 mg[3]	100 mg PO equivalent to codeine 32 mg PO; accumulation of metabolites can lead to CNS, cardiac and respiratory depression. Convulsions, cardiotoxicity and fatal overdose have occurred.
4-6 hrs	50-100 mg	Weak agonist/norepinephrine and serotonin reuptake inhibitor; variable response and threshold for nausea and vomiting; 50 mg equivalent to codeine 60 mg; 100 mg comparable to aspirin 650 mg plus codeine 60 mg; maximum dose 400 mg/d for IR and 300 mg/d for ER; lowers seizure threshold.
24 hrs	100 mg	
4-6 hrs	50-100 mg	Weak mu-receptor agonist, norepinephrine reuptake inhibitor. A new medication with fewer GI adverse effects, but similar CNS effects compared to other weak opioid agonists. Less potent than morphine.

Continued on next page.

SOME OPIOID ANALGESICS (continued)

Drug
PARTIAL AGONISTS AND MIXED AGONIST/ANTAGONISTS
Buprenorphine
Buprenex (Reckitt Benckiser)
Butorphanol
Stadol (Novartis)
Nalbuphine
Pentazocine
Talwin (Hospira)

(Abstral), a nasal spray *(Lazanda)* and a sublingual spray *(Subsys)* for management of breakthrough pain in cancer patients.

METHADONE — Methadone is used parenterally and orally for treatment of chronic nociceptive pain. It may also be effective for neuropathic pain.[18-20] In one study of first-line treatment of cancer pain, methadone was similar to long-acting morphine.[21] Since the plasma half-life of methadone is variable and can be as long as 5 days, repeated doses can lead to accumulation and CNS depression if used without close monitoring during the

Duration of Action	Starting Oral Dose	Comments
4-6 hrs	—	Partial agonist; virtually no psychotomimetic effects; not available PO for pain; available as sublingual tablets alone (*Subutex*, and others) or with naloxone *(Suboxone)* for treatment of opioid dependence. Also available in a transdermal patch *(Butrans)* for treatment of moderate to severe chronic pain.
3-6 hrs	—	Mixed agonist/antagonist. Not available orally.
3-6 hrs	—	Mixed agonist/antagonist; fewer psychotomimetic effects than pentazocine. Not available orally.
2-4 hrs	—	Mixed agonist/antagonist; 50 mg PO equivalent to codeine 60 mg PO; highly irritating to tissues; psychotomimetic effects; available orally only in combinations with acetaminophen or naloxone (to discourage abuse).

titration period. Methadone is not fully cross-tolerant with other opioid agonists. Switiching from another opioid agonist to methadone should be done cautiously; the equianalgesic dose of methadone is not well established in opioid-tolerant patients. Methadone has no active metabolites, which may be advantageous in patients with renal insufficiency. Dose-related QT interval prolongation, torsades de pointes and death have been reported with methadone[22]; a pre-treatment EKG and follow-up at 30 days and then annually are recommended.[23]

Drugs for Pain

LEVORPHANOL — Like methadone, levorphanol is used parenterally and orally to treat chronic pain. It also has a long half-life (16-18 hours) and can accumulate with repeated dosing.

MEPERIDINE — Meperidine should be used only for short-term (24-48 hours) treatment of moderate to severe acute pain. It has a more rapid onset of action than morphine, but it is shorter acting and, when given subcutaneously, highly irritating to tissues. Given IM, repeated doses can cause muscle fibrosis. Repeated doses of the drug lead to accumulation of normeperidine, a toxic metabolite with a 15- to 30-hour half-life. Normeperidine can cause dysphoria, irritability, tremors, myoclonus and, occasionally, seizures, particularly with impaired renal function, use in the elderly or patient-controlled analgesia.[24] In patients taking a monoamine oxidase inhibitor, meperidine can cause severe encephalopathy and death.

WEAK AGONIST/REUPTAKE INHIBITOR — **Tapentadol** *(Nucynta)* is an oral mu-opioid receptor agonist and a norepinephrine reuptake inhibitor. Due to its adrenergic effects, tapentadol should not be used with or within 14 days of a monoamine oxidase inhibitor. Although it does not appear to have significant serotonergic activity, the drug's labeling carries a warning about the possibility of causing serotonin syndrome when used concurrently with serotonergic drugs. Tapentadol is classified as a Schedule II controlled substance and, like other mu agonists, has the potential for addiction and abuse.[25]

Tramadol, an oral centrally-acting opioid agonist that blocks reuptake of norepinephrine and serotonin, is marketed for treatment of moderate to moderately severe pain. It has also been effective for treatment of neuropathic pain in controlled clinical trials.[26] Tramadol's effectiveness in combination with acetaminophen is comparable to that of combinations of aspirin or acetaminophen with codeine or propoxyphene. Seizures have been reported with tramadol; patients with a history of seizures and those concomitantly taking a tricyclic or selective serotonin reuptake

SOME OPIOID COMBINATIONS

Drugs	Strengths (mg)
Acetaminophen-containing	
Codeine/acetaminophen *Tylenol w/codeine no. 3*, others	30/300, 60/300
Hydrocodone/acetaminophen *Vicodin, Lortab*, others	7.5/300, 5/300, 10/300, 5/325, 7.5/325, 10/325, 5/400, 7.5/400,10/400, 2.5/500, 5/500, 7.5/500, 10/500, 7.5/650, 10/650, 10/660, 7.5/750,10/750
Oxycodone/acetaminophen *Percocet, Roxicet*, others	2.5/300, 5/300, 7.5/300, 10/300, 2.5/400, 5/400, 7.5/400, 10/400, 2.5/325, 5/325, 7.5/325,10/325, 5/500, 7.5/500, 10/500, 10/650
Pentazocine/acetaminophen *Talacen*, others	25/650
Propoxyphene HCl*/acetaminophen *Darvocet*	65/650
Propoxyphene napsylate*/ acetaminophen *Darvocet N*	50/325, 100/500, 100/650
Tramadol/acetaminophen *Ultracet*, others	37.5/325
Aspirin-containing	
Oxycodone/aspirin *Percodan*, others	5/325
Ibuprofen-containing	
Hydrocodone/ibuprofen *Reprexain, Vicoprofen*, others	5/200, 7.5/200, 10/200
Oxycodone/ibuprofen *Combunox*	5/400

*Products containing propoxyphene are no longer available in the US.

EQUIANALGESIC DOSES OF SOME OPIOID AGONISTS*

Drug	Route	Dose Approximately Equivalent to 10 mg IM Morphine
Strong Full Agonists		
Fentanyl	IM	0.1 mg
	TD	0.2 mg
	TM	0.2 mg
Hydromorphone	IM	1.5 mg
	PO	7.5 mg
Levorphanol	SC	2 mg (single dose)
		1 mg (chronic pain)
	PO	4 mg (single dose)
		1 mg (chronic pain)
Meperidine	IM	75-100 mg
	PO	300 mg
Methadone	IM	10 mg (single dose)
		1 mg (chronic pain)
	PO	20 mg (single dose)
		2 mg (chronic pain)
Morphine	IM	10 mg
	PO	30 mg
Oxycodone	PO	15-20 mg
Oxymorphone	IM	1 mg
	PO	10 mg
Partial Agonists and Mixed Agonist/Antagonists		
Buprenorphine	IM	0.4 mg
Butorphanol	IM	2 mg
Nalbuphine	IM	10 mg
Pentazocine	IM	30 mg
	PO	50 mg

* When switching from one opioid to another, half the equianalgesic dose should be used initially, and then retitrated.
TD = transdermal; TM = transmucosal

inhibitor (SSRI) antidepressant, an MAO inhibitor, other opioids or an antipsychotic drug may be at increased risk. The need for slow-dose titration when initiating tramadol limits its use for the treatment of acute pain. Tramadol is not scheduled as a controlled substance, but psychological and physical dependence have occurred. Dosages of tramadol should not exceed 400 mg per day.

PARTIAL AGONISTS AND MIXED AGONIST/ANTAGONISTS — This group includes the partial agonist **buprenorphine** and the mixed agonist/antagonists **pentazocine**, **butorphanol** and **nalbuphine**. All of these drugs have a ceiling on their analgesic effects and can precipitate withdrawal symptoms in patients physically dependent on full agonists. All are less likely than full agonists to cause physical dependence, but none is entirely free of dependence liability. They can all be given parenterally, but pentazocine is too irritating to tissues for continued parenteral use. Pentazocine is also available for oral use, but only in combination products. Buprenorphine is available orally as sublingual tablets and in combination with naloxone for treatment of opioid dependence.[27] It is also available for parenteral use.

TOLERANCE TO OPIOIDS — Tolerance can develop with chronic use of opioids[28]; the patient first notices a reduction in adverse effects and a shorter duration of analgesia followed by a decrease in the effectiveness of each dose. Tolerance develops to most of the adverse effects of opioids at least as rapidly as tolerance to the analgesic effect. It can, therefore, usually be surmounted and adequate analgesia restored by increasing the dose. Cross-tolerance exists among all full agonists, but is not complete; when switching to another opioid, starting with half of the customary equianalgesic dose is recommended. Switching opioid-tolerant patients to methadone may improve pain relief.

PHYSICAL DEPENDENCE — Patients being treated with opioids will develop physical dependence with abstinence symptoms if the drug is discontinued suddenly or an opioid antagonist is given. Clinically significant dependence develops only after several weeks of chronic treatment with any dose of an opioid.

Addiction is characterized by impaired control over use of the prescribing drug (compulsive behavior) and craving. Some patients may be predisposed to develop addictive behavior when exposed to opioids.

OPIOID-INDUCED HYPERALGESIA — Opioid-induced hyperalgesia is a controversial condition in which patients treated with high doses of opioids experience worsening pain that cannot be overcome simply by increasing the dose (as is the case in tolerance), but rather only by completely discontinuing the opioid, reducing the dose or changing to an alternate opioid.[29]

ADVERSE EFFECTS — Sedation, dizziness, nausea, vomiting, itching, sweating and constipation are the most common adverse effects of opioids; respiratory depression is the most serious. Persistent opioid-induced sedation that limits activity can be ameliorated by giving small oral doses of stimulants such as methylphenidate (*Ritalin*, and others) in the morning and early afternoon. The narcolepsy drug modafinil *(Provigil)* has also been shown to be beneficial in opioid-induced sedation.[30] Tolerance usually develops rapidly to the sedative and emetic effects of opioids, but not to constipation; a stimulant laxative with or without a stool softener should be started early in treatment. Transdermal fentanyl may cause less sedation and less constipation than sustained-release oral morphine. The opioid antagonist methylnaltrexone *(Relistor)*, administered subcutaneously, can reverse opioid-induced constipation.[31,32]

In patients with chronic obstructive pulmonary disease, cor pulmonale, decreased respiratory reserve or pre-existing respiratory depression, usual doses of opioids, including the mixed agonist/antagonists, may decrease respiratory drive and cause apnea when given acutely. Although patients without pulmonary disease who take opioids chronically are often tolerant to the respiratory depressant effect, opioid-naive acute-pain patients are far more susceptible and therefore must be closely monitored. The addition of general anesthetics, phenothiazines, sedative-hypnotics such as benzodiazepines and barbiturates, tricyclic antidepressants or other CNS depressants increases the risk of respiratory depression.

DOSAGE — Opioid dose requirements vary widely from one patient to another, but 10 mg of morphine per 70 kg body weight or its equivalent is a reasonable starting dose. There is generally no maximum dose except when limited by the dose of aspirin, acetaminophen or ibuprofen in fixed-dose combination preparations. The dose required to maintain optimum pain relief with tolerable side effects should be used. After initial titration with a short-acting opioid in the first 12-24 hours and determination of the 24-hour dose requirement, around-the-clock dosing is recommended for persistent chronic pain. Rapid-onset opioids in doses that are 10-15% of the total daily dose should be made available every 2-3 hours for breakthrough pain. Patient-controlled analgesia with morphine or hydromorphone, given intravenously, epidurally, transdermally or by other routes, is now also widely used.

AN INTRATHECAL ANALGESIC

Ziconotide *(Prialt)*, a synthetic neuronal N-type calcium channel blocker, is approved by the FDA for treatment of severe chronic pain.[33] It is administered intrathecally via a programmable microinfusion device. Ziconotide has lowered pain scores in some patients as monotherapy and when added to standard therapy for refractory severe chronic pain, including neuropathic pain, but severe psychiatric effects (paranoid reactions, psychosis) and CNS toxicity (confusion, somnolence, unresponsiveness) have occurred. Unlike opioids, ziconotide does not cause tolerance, dependence or respiratory depression, and is not a controlled substance. Both the drug itself and the cost of implanting a spinal infusion pump system are expensive.

ADJUVANT PAIN MEDICATIONS

Antidepressants and anticonvulsants are the mainstay of treatment for a variety of neuropathic pain syndromes, including postherpetic neuralgia, diabetic neuropathy, fibromyalgia, complex regional pain syndrome and phantom limb pain, even though most of them are not approved by the FDA for these indications. Combination use of antidepressant and anticonvulsant medication may produce synergistic increases in analgesic effect in neuropathic pain syndromes.[34]

ANTIDEPRESSANTS — Tricyclic antidepressants such as **amitriptyline** (*Elavil*, and others), **nortriptyline** (*Pamelor*, and others) and **imipramine** (*Tofranil*, and others) can relieve many types of neuropathic pain, including diabetic neuropathy, postherpetic neuralgia, polyneuropathy, and nerve injury or infiltration with cancer. Antidepressants are also effective analgesics in fibromyalgia pain.[35] The analgesic effects of these drugs are thought to come from their inhibition of norepinephrine and serotonin reuptake; antagonism of cholinergic and histaminergic systems is responsible for their adverse effects of sedation, urinary retention and hypotension. SSRIs appear to be less effective than tricyclic antidepressants for treatment of neuropathic pain.[36]

Venlafaxine (*Effexor*, and others), a serotonin and norepinephrine reuptake inhibitor (SNRI), has been reported to be effective in neuropathic pain and has also been used to treat headache, fibromyalgia and postmastectomy pain syndrome.[37] Withdrawal symptoms may be troublesome, however. **Duloxetine** (*Cymbalta*), another SNRI, is approved for treatment of pain associated with diabetic peripheral neuropathy and fibromyalgia.[38,39] It was also recently FDA-approved for treatment of chronic musculoskeletal pain; in studies in patients with chronic low back pain or osteoarthritis, duloxetine was modestly more effective than placebo.[52] Duloxetine appears to provide many of the analgesic benefits of older antidepressants with fewer adverse effects. **Milnacipran** (*Savella*) has been approved by the FDA for use in fibromyalgia.[40] It appears to be moderately effective in decreasing pain and improving function; how it compares to venlafaxine or duloxetine remains to be established.

ANTICONVULSANTS — In controlled trials, **gabapentin** (*Neurontin, Gralise,* and others) has been effective in postherpetic neuralgia (an FDA-approved use) and diabetic neuropathy (off-label).[41] It is also used off-label for other types of neuropathic pain. In one study in patients with postherpetic neuralgia or diabetic neuropathy, gabapentin and morphine combined achieved better analgesia at lower doses of each drug than either as a single agent.[42] Dizziness, somnolence, edema and weight gain can occur. **Pregabalin** (*Lyrica*), which is similar in structure to gabapentin, is approved for treatment of neuropathic pain associated with postherpetic neuralgia and diabetic peripheral neuropathy, and for fibromyalgia. Because of some reports of euphoria, it is a Schedule V controlled substance. Like gabapentin, it can cause dizziness, somnolence and peripheral edema; significant weight gain has been reported in some patients. The dose can be titrated more rapidly than with gabapentin, and pregabalin can be given twice rather than 3 times daily.[43,44] **Carbamazepine** (*Tegretol*, and others) is FDA-approved for treatment of pain due to trigeminal neuralgia. **Oxcarbazepine** (*Trileptal,* and others), which is related to carbamazepine, has been shown to provide similar analgesia with fewer adverse effects. **Lamotrigine** (*Lamictal*, and others) was effective for central post-stroke pain and HIV-associated painful sensory neuropathies in small trials, but larger trials have been less positive. Lamotrigine can cause rash that has sometimes progressed to Stevens-Johnson syndrome. **Sodium valproate** (*Depakote*, and others) and **topiramate** (*Topamax,* and others) have been used for migraine prophylaxis.

OTHERS — **Caffeine** in doses of 65-200 mg may enhance the analgesic effect of acetaminophen, aspirin or ibuprofen. **Hydroxyzine** in doses of 25-50 mg given parenterally may add to the analgesic effect of opioids in postoperative and cancer pain while reducing the incidence of nausea and vomiting. **Corticosteroids** can produce analgesia in some patients with inflammatory diseases or tumor infiltration of nerves. The oral and trans-dermal patch formulation of the alpha$_2$-adrenergic agonist **clonidine** (*Catapres*, and others) may improve pain and hyperalgesia in sympatheti-cally maintained pain. **Botulinum** toxin type A adminstered intradermally appeared to be effective in one study for diabetic peripheral neuropathy pain.[54] Although controversial, medical marijuana has been shown to be effective in multiple sclerosis patients with central neuropathic pain; data supporting its efficacy for intractable cancer pain are limited.[46]

Topical analgesics are generally safe and well tolerated. A 5% lidocaine patch *(Lidoderm)* was approved by the FDA for treatment of postherpetic neuralgia.[47] Topical *EMLA*, a mixture of the local anesthetics lidocaine and prilocaine, is useful for cutaneous anesthesia.[48] A formulation of lidocaine and tetracaine in patch form *(Synera)* is approved for anesthesia before acute topical procedures such as venipuncture. A diclofenac patch *(Flector)* has been approved by the FDA for local treatment of muscu-loskeletal pain.[49] An 8% capsaicin patch *(Qutenza)* has been approved for treatment of postherpetic neuralgia.[53] A diclofenac topical gel *(Voltaren 1% Gel)* has been approved for treatment of osteoarthritis in knees and hands.

SUMMARY

The nonopioid analgesics aspirin, acetaminophen and NSAIDs are pre-ferred for initial treatment of mild to moderate pain. In single full doses, most NSAIDs are more effective analgesics than full doses of aspirin or acetaminophen for moderate pain, and some have shown equal or greater analgesic effect than usual doses of an oral opioid combined with acetaminophen, or even injected opioids. The selective COX-2 inhibitor celecoxib appears to cause less severe GI toxicity than non-selective NSAIDs. Moderate pain that does not respond to nonopioids can be treated with weak opioids combined with nonopioid analgesics. Care must be taken when prescribing combination drugs containing acetaminophen and opioids not to give an inappropriately high dose of acetaminophen when titrating the opioid to a therapeutic level.[50]

For treatment of most types of severe pain (some severe neuropathic pain may respond to nonopioids), strong full opioid agonists are the drugs of choice. Unlike NSAIDs, morphine and the other full agonists generally have no ceiling for their analgesic effectiveness except that imposed by adverse effects. Morphine is the standard of comparison, but patients who do not respond to one opioid may respond to another. Meperidine use should be discouraged because of the high rate of CNS toxicity and the availability of less toxic, longer-acting alternatives. Tolerance to most of the adverse effects of opioids, including respiratory and CNS depression, develops at least as rapidly as tolerance to the analgesic effect; tolerance can, therefore, usually be surmounted and adequate analgesia restored by increasing the dose. When frequent dosing becomes impractical, long-acting opioids may be helpful. Combination regimens using nonopioids, opioids and adjuvant analgesics can be useful for severe chronic pain such as occurs in cancer patients.

1. ED Belay et al. Reye's syndrome in the United States from 1981 through 1997. N Engl J Med 1999; 340:1377.
2. PB Watkins et al. Aminotransferase elevations in healthy adults receiving 4 grams of acetaminophen daily: a randomized controlled trial. JAMA 2006; 296:87.
3. Medical Letter Adverse Drug Interactions Program.
4. J Bannwarth et al. Single and multiple dose pharmacokinetics of acetaminophen (paracetamol) in polymedicated very old patients with rheumatic pain. J Rheumatol 2001; 28:182.
5. Primary prevention of ulcers in patients taking aspirin or NSAIDs. Med Lett Drugs Ther 2010; 52:17.
6. Intravenous ibuprofen (Caldolor). Med Lett Drugs Ther 2010; 52:3.
7. Celecoxib for arthritis. Med Lett Drugs Ther 1999; 41:11.
8. JR Caldwell et al. Efficacy and safety of a once-daily morphine formulation in chronic, moderate-to-severe osteoarthritis pain: results from a randomized, placebo-controlled, double-blind trial and an open-label extension trial. J Pain Symptom Manage 2002; 23:278.
9. A morphine.naltrexone combination (Embeda) for analgesia. Med Lett Drugs Ther 2010; 52:22.

Drugs for Pain

10. CM Reid et al. Oxycodone for cancer-related pain: meta-analysis of randomized controlled trials. Arch Intern Med 2006; 166:837.
11. Oral oxymorphone (Opana). Med Lett Drugs Ther 2007; 49:3.
12. PA Sloan and R Barkin. Oxymorphone and oxymorphone extended release: a pharmacotherapeutic review. J Opioid Manag 2008; 4:131.
13. In brief: heat and transdermal fentanyl. Med Lett Drugs Ther 2009; 51:64.
14. CYP3A and drug interactions. Med Lett Drugs Ther 2005; 47:54.
15. RK Portenoy et al. Fentanyl buccal tablet (FBT) for relief of breakthrough pain in opioid-treated patients with chronic low back pain: a randomized, placebo-controlled study. Curr Med Res Opin 2007; 23:223.
16. M Darwish et al. Absolute and relative bioavailability of fentanyl buccal tablet and oral transmucosal fentanyl citrate. J Clin Pharmacol 2007; 47:343.
17. Fentanyl buccal tablet (Fentora) for breakthrough pain. Med Lett Drugs Ther 2007; 49:79.
18. JS Morley et al. Low-dose methadone has an analgesic effect in neuropathic pain: a double-blind randomized controlled crossover trial. Palliat Med 2003; 17:576.
19. MC Rowbotham et al. Oral opioid therapy for chronic peripheral and central neuropathic pain. N Engl J Med 2003; 348:1223.
20. KM Foley. Opioids and chronic neuropathic pain. N Engl J Med 2003; 348:1279.
21. E Bruera et al. Methadone versus morphine as a first-line strong opioid for cancer pain: a randomized, double-blind study. J Clin Oncol 2004; 22:185.
22. GB Ehret et al. Drug-induced long QT syndrome in injection drug users receiving methadone: high frequency in hospitalized patients and risk factors. Arch Intern Med 2006; 166:1280.
23. MJ Krantz et al. QTc interval screening in methadone treatment. Ann Intern Med 2009; 150:387.
24. CF Seifert and S Kennedy. Meperidine is alive and well in the new millennium: evaluation of meperidine usage patterns and frequency of adverse drug reactions. Pharmacotherapy 2004; 24:776.
25. Tapentadol (Nucynta) – a new analgesic. Med Lett Drugs Ther 2009; 51:61.
26. RM Duehmke et al. Tramadol for neuropathic pain (review). Cochrane Database Syst Rev 2004; (2):CD003726.
27. Buprenorphine: an alternative to methadone. Med Lett Drugs Ther 2003; 45:13.
28. P Sloan and N Babul. Extended-release opioids for the management of chronic non-malignant pain. Expert Opin Drug Deliv 2006; 3:489.
29. K Bannister and AH Dickenson. Opioid hyperalgesia. Curr Opin Support Palliat Care 2010; 4:1.
30. New indications for modafinil (Provigil). Med Lett Drugs Ther 2004; 46:34.
31. Methylnaltrexone (Relistor) for opioid-induced constipation. Med Lett Drugs Ther 2008; 50:63.
32. J Thomas et al. Methylnaltrexone for opioid-induced constipation in advanced illness. N Engl J Med 2008; 358:2332.
33. Ziconotide (Prialt) for chronic pain. Med Lett Drugs Ther 2005; 47:103.
34. I Gilron et al. Nortriptyline and gabapentin, alone and in combination for neuropathic pain: a double-blind, randomised controlled crossover trial. Lancet 2009; 374:1252.

35. W Hauser et al. Treatment of fibromyalgia syndrome with antidepressants: a meta-analysis. JAMA 2009; 301:198.
36. SH Sindrup et al. Antidepressants in the treatment of neuropathic pain. Basic Clin Pharmacol Toxicol 2005; 96:399.
37. DR Grothe et al. Treatment of pain syndromes with venlafaxine. Pharmacotherapy 2004; 24:621.
38. Duloxetine (Cymbalta) for diabetic neuropathic pain. Med Lett Drugs Ther 2005; 47:67.
39. Duloxetine (Cymbalta) for fibromyalgia. Med Lett Drugs Ther 2008; 50:57.
40. Milnacipran (Savella) for fibromyalgia. Med Lett Drugs Ther 2009; 51:45.
41. Gabapentin (Neurontin) for chronic pain. Med Lett Drugs Ther 2004; 46:29.
42. I Gilron et al. Morphine, gabapentin, or their combination for neuropathic pain. N Engl J Med 2005; 352:1324.
43. Pregabalin (Lyrica) for neuropathic pain and epilepsy. Med Lett Drugs Ther 2005; 47:75.
44. W Hauser et al. Treatment of fibromyalgia syndrome with gabapentin and pregabalin—a meta-analysis of randomized controlled trials. Pain 2009; 145:69.
45. RY Yuan et al. Botulinum toxin for diabetic neuropathic pain: a randomized double-blind crossover trial. Neurology 2009; 72:1473.
46. Medical marijuana. Med Lett Drugs Ther 2010; 52:5.
47. PS Davies and BS Galer. Review of lidocaine patch 5% studies in the treatment of postherpetic neuralgia. Drugs 2004; 64:937.
48. V Lindh et al. EMLA cream and oral glucose for immunization pain in 3-month-old infants. Pain 2003; 104:381.
49. A diclofenac patch (Flector) for pain. Med Lett Drugs Ther 2008; 50:1.
50. Acetaminophen safety – déjà vu. Med Lett Drugs Ther 2009; 51:53.
51. Intravenous acetaminophen (Ofirmev). Med Lett Drugs Ther 2011; 53:26.
52. Duloxetine (Cymbalta) for chronic musculoskeletal pain. Med Lett Drugs Ther 2011; 53:33.
53. Capsaicin patch (Qutenza) for postherpetic neuralgia. Med Lett Drugs Ther 2011; 53:42.

DOES ACETAMINOPHEN INCREASE BLOOD PRESSURE?

Originally published in The Medical Letter – April 2011; 53:29

A recent article in *Circulation* reported that acetaminophen (*Tylenol*, and others; paracetamol outside the US) increased blood pressure in patients with coronary artery disease. This conclusion was based on a randomized, placebo-controlled crossover trial in 33 patients; acetaminophen 1 g three times daily for 2 weeks was associated with statistically significant increases in blood pressure of 2.9 mmHg systolic and 2.2 mmHg diastolic.[1]

NSAIDs can increase blood pressure; the mechanism is thought to be inhibition of cyclooxygenase leading to decreased renal prostaglandin activity. Acetaminophen also inhibits cyclooxygenase (primarily COX-2) and decreases prostaglandin activity.[2]

The small increases in blood pressure reported with acetaminophen would probably be inconsequential in low-risk patients, but might be a concern for those with cardiovascular disease. Like most drugs, acetaminophen should be used in the lowest effective doses for the shortest possible time. Mild to moderate pain due to osteoarthritis or headache generally responds to a dose of 650 mg.[3]

1. I Sudano et al. Acetaminophen increases blood pressure in patients with coronary artery disease. Circulation 2010; 122:1789.
2. B Hinz et al. Acetaminophen (paracetamol) is a selective cyclooxygenase-2 inhibitor in man. FASEB J 2008; 22:383.
3. Drugs for pain. Treat Guidel Med Lett 2010; 8:25.

EPIDURAL CORTICOSTEROID INJECTIONS FOR LUMBAR AND CERVICAL RADICULOPATHY

Originally published in The Medical Letter – January 2012; 54:5

For patients with radicular pain unresponsive to conservative treatment after 1-2 months and no progressive neurologic deficit, epidural corticosteroid injections are often tried before surgical intervention.

CLINICAL STUDIES — Published studies of corticosteroid injections for radiculopathy have usually been small and short-term, used various corticosteroids in different doses and fluid volumes, included and excluded patients with various etiologies, and used a variety of endpoints to measure outcomes. Some studies used placebo controls; most did not. A few studies were randomized; none were double-blind.

Lumbar Radiculopathy – One review found strong evidence that use of lumbar epidural steroid injections produced short-term relief of unilateral radicular pain caused by herniated nucleus pulposus or spinal stenosis.[1] A review of studies using only a transforaminal (rather than an interlaminar) approach found strong evidence for short-term relief and moderate evidence for long-term relief of radicular pain caused by impingement or stenosis.[2] A third review that included both interlaminar and transforaminal approaches found a moderate short-term benefit in patients with disc herniation and radiculitis.[3]

In contrast, 3 randomized controlled trials of transforaminal epidural steroid injections for lumbar radicular pain that followed patients for 3 months or longer found no benefit.[4]

Cervical Radiculopathy – A prospective study of 68 patients entered over a 10-year period with an average duration of cervical radiculopathy symptoms of 2 months at entry found that after an average follow-up of 39 months, serial cervical injections (an average of 2.5 injections) resolved symptoms in all patients.[5] A retrospective study of 76 patients with neck pain and radiculopathy found that a single cervical epidural injection relieved pain within 2 weeks in 72% of patients (86% of those with a herniated disk and 60% with spinal stenosis).[6] A study of 159 patients entered over a 2-year period who had transforaminal cervical injections found that within 1 month, the treatment was effective in 76% of patients.[7]

In contrast, a controlled trial in 40 patients with cervical radiculopathy randomized to receive injections either with mepivacaine plus methyl-prednisolone acetate or with mepivacaine plus saline solution found no significant difference in treatment results after 3 weeks' follow-up.[8]

ADVERSE EFFECTS — Lumbar steroid injections are generally well tolerated, but one review found that dural puncture, which can cause headache, nausea and vertigo, occurred in 2-5% of procedures. When dural puncture leads to subdural injection of the corticosteroid with its buffer and preservatives, more serious injuries can occur. Twelve cases of paraplegia immediately following lumbar injections have been reported since 2002; most of these patients had had previous surgery in or around the site of injection.[3]

Cervical steroid injections are also generally well tolerated, but major complications of interlaminar cervical steroid injections have rarely included permanent spinal cord injury.[9] Major complications of cervical transforaminal injections have included brain and spinal cord infarction; in one published report, 15 of 105 complications led to death.[10]

CONCLUSION — Both cervical and lumbar epidural corticosteroid injections are generally well tolerated and can be effective in providing short-term relief of pain associated with radiculopathy, and possibly long-term relief in some patients. Rarely, they can cause serious adverse effects, including paraplegia with lumbar injections and brain infarction with cervical injections.

1. ME Rho and CT Tang. The efficacy of lumbar epidural steroid injections: transforaminal, interlaminar, and caudal approaches. Phys Med Rehabil Clin N Am 2011; 22:139.
2. B Benny and P Azari. The efficacy of lumbosacral transforaminal epidural steroid injections: a comprehensive literature review. J Back Musculoskelet Rehabil 2011; 24:67.

3. M Benoist et al. Epidural steroid injections in the management of low-back pain with radiculopathy: an update of their efficacy and safety. Eur Spine J 2011Sep 16 (epub).
4. NA Quraishi. Transforaminal injection of corticosteroids for lumbar radiculopathy: systematic review and meta-analysis. Eur Spine J 2011 Sept 4 (epub).
5. K Bush and S Hillier. Outcome of cervical radiculopathy treated with periradicular/epidural corticosteroid injections: a prospective study with independent clinical review. Eur Spine J 1996; 5:319.
6. JW Kwon et al. Cervical interlaminar epidural steroid injection for neck pain and cervical radiculopathy: effect and prognostic factors. Skeletal Radiol 2007; 36:431.
7. JW Lee et al. Cervical transforaminal epidural steroid injection for the management of cervical radiculopathy: a comparative study of particulate versus non-particulate steroids. Skeletal Radiol 2009; 38:1077.
8. L Anderberg et al. Transforaminal steroid injections for the treatment of cervical radiculopathy: a prospective and randomised study. Eur Spine J 2007; 16:321.
9. A Abbasi et al. Complications of interlaminar cervical epidural steroid injections: a review of the literature. Spine 2007; 32:2144.
10. B Benny et al. Complications of cervical transforaminal epidural steroid injections. Am J Phys Med Rehabil 2010; 89:601.

DRUGS FOR
Parkinson's Disease

Original publication date – January 2011

Parkinson's disease (PD) is caused primarily by progressive degeneration of dopamine-containing neurons in the substantia nigra. Dopamine itself cannot be used to treat PD because it does not cross the blood-brain barrier.

LEVODOPA — Levodopa, the immediate precursor of dopamine, is decarboxylated to dopamine in both brain and peripheral tissues. The combination of levodopa with carbidopa, a peripheral decarboxylase inhibitor, is the most effective treatment available for symptomatic relief of PD.

Limitations – For the first 2-5 years of treatment, levodopa produces a sustained response, but as the disease progresses, the duration of benefit from each dose becomes shorter (the "wearing-off" effect), and still later some patients develop sudden, unpredictable fluctuations between mobility and immobility (the "on-off" effect). After about 5-8 years, the majority of patients have dose-related clinical fluctuations and dose-related dyskinesias (chorea, dystonia). As the disease progresses, levodopa-resistant motor problems including difficulties with balance, gait, speech and swallowing and non-motor symptoms including autonomic, cognitive and psychiatric difficulties become more prominent.

Drugs for Parkinson's Disease

Adverse Effects – While *in vitro* levodopa can be a potent neurotoxin and damage dopaminergic cells,[1] there is no convincing clinical evidence suggesting a toxic effect of the drug in Parkinson's disease. Peripheral adverse effects of levodopa, including anorexia, nausea, vomiting and orthostatic hypotension, are prominent at the beginning of levodopa therapy. With chronic therapy, vivid dreams, hallucinations, delusions, confusion and agitation can occur, especially in older patients with dementia. Pathologic gambling (which is more common with dopamine agonists), compulsive shopping, binge eating, hypersexual behavior, or compulsive repetitive behaviors such as endless writing, singing or talking have also been associated with levodopa therapy.[2,3] Concerns that levodopa and other dopamine agonists could increase the risk of melanoma appear to be unfounded; patients with PD, regardless of treatment, have twice the general incidence of melanoma.[4]

Sudden discontinuation or abrupt reduction of levodopa dosage for several days may cause a severe return of parkinsonian symptoms.

Dosage – The half-life of levodopa when given with carbidopa is only 60-90 minutes. The daily dosage range of levodopa is usually 300-1500 mg divided into 3 to 6 doses; some patients, such as those who develop "wearing-off" phenomena, may require more frequent or higher dosing. Dietary protein may decrease the effectiveness of levodopa by competing with the drug for absorption from the intestine and transport across the blood-brain barrier.

Relatively complete inhibition of peripheral dopa decarboxylase requires 75-100 mg/day of carbidopa; some patients require doses of up to 200 mg/day to completely suppress nausea. Carbidopa *(Lodosyn)* is available alone in doses of 25 mg and can be added to carbidopa/levodopa.

Carbidopa/levodopa is available in immediate- and sustained-release tablets *(Sinemet, Sinemet CR,* and others) and in orally disintegrating tablets *(Parcopa)* that can be taken without liquid.[5] Some clinicians have used "liquid (dissolved) levodopa," chewed or crushed tablets mixed with a carbonated beverage for rapid absorption, as rescue treatment for "off" episodes.[6]

Sustained-release formulations may be beneficial for patients who have "wearing-off" phenomena, but they can be erratically absorbed and have a slower and less predictable onset of action. Many patients must take a half or a whole immediate-release (IR) carbidopa/levodopa tablet concomitantly with sustained-release (CR) preparations, particularly with the first dose of the day. Because only about 70% of levodopa is absorbed from this formulation, the dosage needs to be about 30% higher than that of the IR form of the combination to achieve a comparable effect. Some clinicians use the CR formulation instead of the IR tablets when introducing the drug, starting with 25/100 mg bid or tid and increasing gradually to 50/200 mg bid, tid or qid.

Strategy – Most clinicians now prefer to start therapy with another drug, particularly in younger patients, who are most prone to develop fluctuations and dyskinesias from levodopa.

DOPAMINE AGONISTS — Dopamine agonists are less effective than levodopa for motor symptoms of PD, but are less likely to cause dyskinesias or motor fluctuations. Used as an adjunct to levodopa in advanced disease, they may permit a reduction in levodopa dosage. Two oral non-ergot dopamine agonists, pramipexole (*Mirapex*, and others) and ropinirole (*Requip*, and others), are widely used for treatment of both early (as monotherapy) and advanced disease (with levodopa). Rotigotine *(Neupro)*, another non-ergot dopamine agonist, is available in a transdermal formulation in Canada and many European countries. In the US, rotigotine was recalled in 2008 because of crystal formation in the patch. Only one ergot-derivative dopamine agonist, bromocriptine (*Parlodel*, and others), is still marketed in the US; pergolide (*Permax*, and others) was taken off the market because its use was associated with cardiac-valve regurgitation.[7,8]

Drugs for Parkinson's Disease

SOME DRUGS FOR PARKINSON'S DISEASE

Drug	Formulations
CARBIDOPA/LEVODOPA	
immediate-release (IR) tablets	10/100 mg, 25/100 mg,
generic	25/250 mg
Sinemet (Bristol-Myers Squibb)	
orally-disintegrating IR tablets	10/100 mg, 25/100 mg,
Parcopa (Schwarz)	25/250 mg
sustained-release tablets – generic	25/100 mg, 50/200 mg
Sinemet CR (Bristol-Myers Squibb)	
DOPAMINE AGONISTS	
Oral	
Bromocriptine – generic	2.5 mg tabs, 5 mg caps
Parlodel (Novartis)	
Pramipexole – generic	0.125, 0.25, 0.5, 0.75,
Mirapex (Boehringer-Ingelheim)	1, 1.5 mg tabs
extended-release tablets	
Mirapex ER	0.375, 0.75, 1.5, 3, 4.5 mg tabs
Ropinirole – generic	0.25, 0.5, 1, 2, 3, 4, 5 mg tabs
Requip (GlaxoSmithKline)	
extended-release tablets	
Requip XL	2, 4, 6, 8, 12mg
Subcutaneous	
Apomorphine – *Apokyn* (Ipsen)	30 mg/3 mL cartridge
COMT INHIBITORS	
Entacapone – *Comtan* (Novartis)	200 mg tabs
Tolcapone – *Tasmar* (Roche)	100, 200 mg tabs
MAO-B INHIBITORS	
Rasagiline – *Azilect* (Teva)	0.5, 1 mg tabs
Selegiline – generic	5 mg tabs, caps
Eldepryl (Somerset)	5 mg caps
orally-disintegrating tablets	
Zelapar (Valeant)	1.25 mg tabs

1. Always administered with levodopa/carbidopa.

Usual Daily Dosage

300-1500 mg levodopa, divided

300-1500 mg levodopa, divided

400-2200 mg levodopa, divided

15 to 45 mg divided bid or tid

0.5 to 1.5 mg tid

1.5-4.5 mg daily
3 to 8 mg tid

8-24 mg daily

2-6 mg SC 3-5x/day prn

200 mg tid or qid[1]
100 mg tid[1]

0.5-1 mg daily
5 mg bid at breakfast and lunch

1.25 to 2.5 mg in the morning

Continued on next page.

Drugs for Parkinson's Disease

SOME DRUGS FOR PARKINSON'S DISEASE (continued)

Drug	Formulations
COMBINATIONS	
Carbidopa/levodopa/entacapone	
Stalevo 50 (Novartis)	12.5/50/200 mg tabs
Stalveo 75	18.75/75/200 mg tabs
Stalevo 100	25/100/200 mg tabs
Stalevo 125	31.25/125/200 mg tabs
Stalevo 150	37.5/150/200 mg tabs
Stalevo 200	50/200/200 mg tabs
OTHER DRUGS	
Amantadine – generic	100 mg caps; 100 mg tabs; 50 mg/5 mL syrup
Carbidopa – *Lodosyn* (Bristol-Myers Squibb)	25 mg tabs

Effectiveness – All of these drugs are effective in early, mild disease, but most patients started on dopamine agonists require addition of levodopa over time.[9] They are also effective when used as add-on treatment in patients with levodopa-induced motor fluctuations.

Dosage – Pramipexole should be started at 0.125 mg tid and gradually increased to 0.75 mg tid over 4-6 weeks. Further increases should be slower, up to an FDA-approved maximum daily dosage of 4.5 mg, but some studies have found no additional efficacy and an increase in adverse effects at doses higher than 1.0-1.5 mg/day. Ropinirole should be started at 0.25 mg tid and slowly titrated up by 0.25 mg or 0.5 mg per dose each week, up to 3 mg or 4 mg tid. Many patients will need to continue gradually increasing the dose to a maximum of 8 mg tid. Both ropinirole and pramipexole are available as controlled-release formulations that can be taken once daily. The recommended initial dose of extended-release ropinirole *(Requip XL)* is 2 mg once daily for 1-2 weeks. The dose can be

Usual Daily Dosage
300-1200 mg levodopa, divided (max 8 tabs)
100 mg bid
25 mg tid or qid

increased at week 1 (or longer intervals) by 2 mg/day increments to a maximum daily dose of 24 mg. Extended-release pramipexole *(Mirapex ER)* is usually started at a dose of 0.375 mg daily. The dose is slowly titrated with weekly (or even slower) increases first to 0.75 mg per day and then by 0.75 mg increments up to a maximum of 4.5 mg per day.

Adverse Effects – Dopamine agonists can cause nausea, somnolence, lower-extremity edema and postural hypotension, which may limit their use. In a controlled trial of pramipexole vs. levodopa for initial therapy, the dopamine agonist caused a higher incidence of somnolence, edema and (most significantly) hallucinations than levodopa did.[10] Sudden sleep attacks can occur with dopamine agonists alone or in combination with levodopa. Rather than sacrifice motor performance by reducing the dose or eliminating the dopamine agonist, some experts treat excessive daytime sleepiness with modafinil *(Provigil)* 200 mg once/day after breakfast (not FDA-approved for this indication).

As the dosage of the dopamine agonist increases, levodopa dosage may have to be decreased. Even used alone or in low doses, dopamine agonists can cause confusion and psychosis, particularly in elderly patients. They should generally not be used in patients with dementia. An increasingly recognized and potentially serious adverse effect of dopamine agonists is an impulse-control disorder, manifested by pathologic gambling, excessive shopping, binge eating or hypersexuality,[3,11] which was previously reported with levodopa use.

Peripheral dopaminergic side effects, such as nausea, can be blocked by domperidone (*Motilium*, and others; available in Canada) or ondansetron (*Zofran*, and others). Ergot-type effects such as erythromelalgia, edema, pain and digital spasms in the extremities occur rarely with bromocriptine. Pleural effusions causing sudden onset of shortness of breath and/or cough, which have occurred rarely with bromocriptine, are reversible if the drug is stopped, but fibrotic pulmonary changes and retroperitoneal fibrosis can occur. Application site reactions have occurred with rotigotine.

An Injectable Dopamine Agonist – Apomorphine *(Apokyn)*, a potent non-ergot dopamine agonist, is FDA-approved for treatment of immobility ("off" episodes) in patients with advanced PD.[12] Administered subcutaneously, it causes emesis and must be taken with trimethobenzamide (*Tigan*, and others) 300 mg tid begun 3 days before initial treatment and continued for at least 2 months. Oral domperidone is also effective in preventing emesis. Serotonin receptor antagonists such as ondansetron are contraindicated for use with apomorphine because the combination can cause severe hypotension with loss of consciousness.

Injection-site reactions can occur. Like the oral dopamine agonists, apomorphine can cause nausea, orthostatic hypotension, dyskinesias, confusion, hallucinations and psychosis. Yawning and drowsiness are common. Hypersexuality and increased erections can occur and have been associated with abuse of the drug.

COMT INHIBITORS — Levodopa is metabolized in the periphery by 2 enzymes, dopa decarboxylase and catechol-O-methyl-transferase (COMT). Used in combination with levodopa, drugs that inhibit peripheral or intestinal activity of COMT prolong the half-life of levodopa (without affecting peak serum concentrations) and decrease parkinsonian disability. The combination, can, however, increase dyskinesias; a reduction in levodopa dosage may be required for control. Entacapone *(Comtan)* has been effective in patients with motor fluctuations, resulting in improvement in "off" time, motor scores and levodopa requirements. It has a short half-life and must be taken with each dose of levodopa. Entacapone is available alone and as a carbidopa/levodopa/entacapone combination *(Stalevo)*. Tolcapone *(Tasmar)* is a more potent COMT inhibitor. It was associated with fatal hepatotoxicity in 3 patients and was taken off the market in Canada, but is available in the US for use in patients who have not responded to entacapone.[13,14]

Dosage – The dose of entacapone is 200 mg tid or qid. The initial dose of tolcapone is 100 mg tid which can be increased to a maximum of 200 mg tid; tolcapone should be stopped if there is no benefit at 3 weeks. Both should always be taken with each dose of levodopa/carbidopa.

Adverse Effects – Dyskinesias, nausea, diarrhea (worse with tolcapone) and urine discoloration can occur with both COMT inhibitors. Serious hepatotoxicity has not been reported with entacapone. Use of tolcapone requires patient written consent and hepatic monitoring twice per month for the first 6 months and periodically thereafter. Since these drugs are used in combination with levodopa, the levodopa dose may have to be decreased in patients who develop dyskinesias, nausea or hallucinations. Increased daytime sleepiness and sleep attacks have been reported with entacapone.

MAO-B INHIBITORS — Selegiline (*Eldepryl, Zelapar,* and others), an irreversible inhibitor of monoamine oxidase type B (MAO-B), inhibits catabolism of dopamine in the brain. Selegiline's effect on symptoms is modest, but used as monotherapy in early disease, it can delay initiation of levodopa treatment. Used in addition to levodopa in advanced disease, it can permit use of lower doses of levodopa.[15] Selegiline is available in a conventional tablet or capsule for swallowing and in a lower-dose orally disintegrating tablet formulation *(Zelapar)*. The disintegrating tablet formulation, which is absorbed through the oral mucosa, minimizes first-pass metabolism, increases bioavailability, and reduces serum concentrations of amphetamine metabolites. The initial dose is 1.25 mg in the morning without liquid or food. After 6 weeks, the dose can be increased to a maximum of 2.5 mg once per day.[16] The initial dose of the swallowed formulation is 5 mg once daily with breakfast, which can be increased to 5 mg with breakfast and with lunch.

Rasagiline *(Azilect),* the second MAO-B inhibitor approved for treatment of PD, also appears to be modestly effective when taken alone for early disease or in addition to levodopa/carbidopa in advanced disease.[17] Rasagiline administered early in the course of the disease may help in delaying its progression. In a double-blind, delayed-start trial of rasagiline, patients receiving 1 mg daily of the drug had significantly less disability after 72 weeks than those who received placebo, but those receiving 2-mg doses did not.[18] In advanced disease, improvement in "off" time is similar to that with entacapone.[19] No studies are available comparing rasagiline to selegiline; only rasagaline is approved by the FDA as an adjunct to levodopa for treatment of Parkinson's disease.

Adverse Effects – Nausea and orthostatic hypotension may occur with MAO-B inhibitors. Unlike MAO-A inhibitors used for treatment of depression, MAO-B inhibitors at recommended doses generally do not cause hypertension after ingestion of tyramine-rich foods or with concomitant levodopa therapy. Some manufacturers recommend dietary restrictions. Combined use of MAO-B inhibitors and tricyclic antidepressants, selective serotonin reuptake inhibitors (SSRIs) or meperidine (*Demerol*, and others) has rarely resulted in severe toxicity. Their package inserts also advise against use with dextromethorphan, propoxyphene, tramadol and methadone. MAO-B inhibitors can also increase levodopa adverse effects, particularly dyskinesias and psychosis in elderly patients.

ANTICHOLINERGICS — Anticholinergics, which include trihexyphenidyl (*Artane*, and others), benztropine (*Cogentin*, and others), procyclidine *(Kemadrin)* and biperiden *(Akineton)* in the US and ethopropazine *(Parsitan)* in Canada, are still useful in some patients with PD, especially for treatment of tremor and drooling. Adverse effects include dry mouth, constipation, urinary retention and aggravation of glaucoma. Central nervous system adverse effects, including impaired memory, confusion and hallucinations, are particularly severe in elderly patients, and generally contraindicate use of anticholinergics in this age group. Abrupt discontinuation of any of these drugs can cause severe exacerbation of symptoms.

AMANTADINE — Amantadine, an antiviral drug, acts as an antagonist at N-methyl-D-aspartate (NMDA) receptors. Its precise mechanism of action in PD is unknown. It has been used alone to treat early PD, or as an adjunct in later stages, usually in patients with levodopa-induced dyskinesias.[20] Amantadine may be effective in controlling tremor, which is often resistant to dopaminergic treatment. In some patients, however, the symptomatic benefit of amantadine can last only a few weeks. Nausea, dizziness, insomnia, confusion, hallucinations, peripheral edema and livedo reticularis can occur. Amantadine is excreted primarily unchanged in urine; the dosage must be decreased for patients with renal dysfunction. High serum concentrations of amantadine cause severe psychosis, particularly in the elderly. Amantadine and anticholinergics may have additive adverse effects on mental function. Sudden withdrawal of amantadine may cause severe exacerbation of parkinsonian symptoms or neuroleptic malignant syndrome and acute delirium.

SURGICAL TREATMENT — Surgery should be reserved for PD patients with major dyskinesias or clinical fluctuations on levodopa. Surgery does not help patients who are unresponsive to levodopa. Appropriate candidates for surgery are those whose cognition is relatively intact on full neuropsychological testing. In selected cases, surgery can also be considered for patients with severe and medically refractory tremor.

Deep Brain Stimulation – Deep brain stimulation (DBS) of the subthalamic nucleus or globus pallidus with high-frequency electrical stimuli from implanted electrodes has supplanted ablative surgical procedures and is now the surgical treatment of choice for PD. A randomized trial in 156 patients with advanced PD (disease duration more than 13 years) found DBS of the subthalamic nucleus plus medication more effective than medication alone in reducing levodopa-related motor symptoms and improving mobility and activities of daily living.[21] In another large randomized trial in 255 patients with PD and motor complications, subjects who underwent bilateral DBS of the subthalamic nucleus or globus pallidus had improved motor function, compared to subjects treated medically, but a higher rate of complications, including one death due to cerebral hemorrhage. Subjects who underwent DBS also had lower performance on cognitive testing.[22] A small study in patients with less advanced disease (average duration 6.8 years) and mild to moderate motor fluctuations on levodopa found that patients treated with DBS of the subthalamic nucleus had less "off" time, used lower doses of levodopa and had better quality of life than matched patients treated with drug therapy.[23] When compared with one another, DBS of either subthalamic nucleus or the globus pallidus produced similar improvement in patients with advanced PD.[24,25]

After DBS, improvement permitting reduction in levodopa dosage may be maintained over several years. In general, treated patients show marked improvement in motor function when off medication and improvement in dyskinesia when taking medication. Some symptoms, such as akinesia, speech disturbances, postural stability, freezing of gait and cognitive problems, did not improve with the procedure and continued to become worse. One device system for performing DBS (*Activa* – Medtronic) has been approved by the FDA for use in tremor and advanced PD.

Adverse Effects – Bilateral DBS is relatively safe, but it carries the risks of invasive brain surgery. Adverse effects have included intracranial hemorrhage, hemiparesis, infection, confusion, attention/cognitive deficits, dysarthria and death. Even with successful surgery, decreased verbal fluency and a variety of psychosocial problems have occurred.[26,27] Hardware problems, including lead migration, fracture or malfunction, occur in 5% of patients.[20] Cognitive decline is also common after DBS in patients with pre-existing intellectual impairment and in older subjects.[28]

TREATMENT OF DEPRESSION — Depression commonly accompanies PD and must be treated if the patient is to benefit adequately from antiparkinson drugs. Worsening of Parkinson's symptoms has been reported rarely with an SSRI. Tricyclic antidepressants, especially nortriptyline, may be more effective than an SSRI.[29] Antidepressants may also help the sleep abnormalities commonly found in PD. Electroconvulsive therapy (ECT) may alleviate refractory major depression and transiently improve the underlying parkinsonian symptoms.

TREATMENT OF PSYCHOSIS — Clozapine (*Clozaril*, and others) is a second-generation antipsychotic that does not cause drug-induced parkinsonism and is particularly useful in controlling psychosis associated with levodopa or dopamine agonists. The usual initial dose for levodopa-induced psychosis is 6.25 or 12.5 mg at bedtime, which can be increased gradually until psychosis is controlled. Drowsiness is a common adverse effect. Clozapine has caused agranulocytosis in 0.6% of patients; weekly blood counts are necessary for the first six months, and biweekly thereafter.

Quetiapine *(Seroquel)* is another antipsychotic drug often used for this indication. The usual dosage is 12.5-100 mg daily, typically at bedtime. It does not cause agranulocytosis and does not have anticholinergic effects. Like clozapine, quetiapine causes drowsiness.[30] It can also be used to improve sleep in more severe cases of insomnia.

TREATMENT OF DEMENTIA — The cholinesterase inhibitors donepezil *(Aricept)*, rivastigmine *(Exelon)* and galantamine *(Razadyne)* used to treat Alzheimer's disease may be useful in treating cognitive and behaviorial symptoms in PD patients, but may worsen tremor in some.[31] Of these, rivastigmine is the only FDA-approved drug for dementia in PD. Memantine *(Namenda)*, an NMDA-receptor antagonist, is another drug used to treat dementia;[32] it may be helpful for cognitive impairment and potentially also for an antiparkinson effect, but may also aggravate parkinsonian symptoms.

CHOICE OF TREATMENT — Levodopa combined with carbidopa remains the most effective symptomatic treatment for Parkinson's disease; sustained-release formulations generally are more erratic in their absorption. Dopamine agonists, the next most effective drugs after levodopa in decreasing symptoms, can be used alone before the introduction of levodopa, or as an adjunct to levodopa. Addition of a peripherally-acting COMT inhibitor or an MAO-B inhibitor to levodopa can reduce motor fluctuations in patients with advanced disease. Anticholinergics are rarely used because of their side effects, but can be a useful addition to levodopa for control of tremor and drooling. Quetiapine and clozapine are the best choices for treatment of psychosis. Subcutaneous apomorphine should be available for rescue use in patients with "off" episodes. Bilateral subthalamic deep brain stimulation is an option for patients with more advanced motor fluctuations and intact cognition.

1. AH Schapira et al. Levodopa in the treatment of Parkinson's disease. Eur J Neurol 2009; 16:982.
2. V Voon et al. Prospective prevalence of pathologic gambling and medication association in Parkinson disease. Neurology 2006; 66:1750.
3. WR Galpern and M Stacy. Management of impulse control disorders in Parkinson's disease. Curr Treat Options Neurol 2007; 9:189.
4. R Zanetti and S Rosso. Levodopa and the risk of melanoma. Lancet 2007; 369:257.
5. Parcopa: a rapidly dissolving formulation of carbidopa/levodopa. Med Lett Drugs Ther 2005; 47:12.
6. M Stacy and S Factor. Rapid treatment of "off" episodes: will this change Parkinson's disease therapy? Neurology 2004; 62 suppl4:S1.

7. R Schade et al. Dopamine agonists and the risk of cardiac-valve regurgitation. N Engl J Med 2007; 356:29.
8. R Zanettini et al. Valvular heart disease and the use of dopamine agonists for Parkinson's disease. N Engl J Med 2007; 356:39.
9. JG Nutt and GF Wooten. Clinical practice. Diagnosis and initial management of Parkinson's disease. N Engl J Med 2005; 353:1021.
10. KM Biglan et al. Risk factors for somnolence, edema, and hallucinations in early Parkinson disease. Neurology 2007; 69:187.
11. DA Gallagher et al. Pathological gambling in Parkinson's disease: risk factors and differences from dopamine dysregulation. An analysis of published case series. Mov Disord 2007; 22:1757.
12. Apomorphine (Apokyn) for advanced Parkinson's disease. Med Lett Drugs Ther 2005; 47:7.
13. J Leegwater-Kim and C Waters. Tolcapone in the management of Parkinson's disease. Expert Opin Pharmacother 2006; 7:2263.
14. Entacapone to Tolcapone Switch Study Investigators. Entacapone to tolcapone switch: Multicenter double-blind, randomized, active-controlled trial in advanced Parkinson's disease. Mov Disord 2007; 22:14.
15. S Pålhagen et al. Selegiline slows the progression of the symptoms of Parkinson disease. Neurology 2006; 66:1200.
16. MF Lew. Selegiline orally disintegrating tablets for the treatment of Parkinson's disease. Expert Rev Neurotherapeutics 2005; 5:705.
17. Rasagiline (Azilect) for Parkinson's disease. Med Lett Drugs Ther 2006; 48:97.
18. CW Olanow et al. ADAGIO Study Investigators: A double-blind, delayed-start trial of rasagiline in Parkinson's disease. N Engl J Med 2009; 361:1268.
19. O Rascol et al. Rasagiline as an adjunct to levodopa in patients with Parkinson's disease and motor fluctuations (LARGO, Lasting effect in Adjunct therapy with Rasagiline Given Once daily, study): a randomised, double-blind, parallel-group trial. Lancet 2005; 365:947.
20. R Pahwa et al. Practice parameter: treatment of Parkinson disease with motor fluctuations and dyskinesia (an evidence-based review): report of the Quality Standards Subcommittee of the American Academy of Neurology. Neurology 2006; 66:983.
21. G Deuschl et al. A randomized trial of deep-brain stimulation for Parkinson's disease. N Engl J Med 2006; 355:896.
22. FM Weaver et al. Bilateral deep brain stimulation vs best medical therapy for patients with advanced Parkinson disease: a randomized controlled trial. JAMA 2009; 301:63.
23. WM Schüpbach et al. Neurosurgery at an earlier stage of Parkinson disease: a randomized, controlled trial. Neurology 2007; 68:267.
24. MS Okun et al. Cognition and mood in Parkinson's disease in subthalamic nucleus versus globus pallidus interna deep brain stimulation: the COMPARE trial. Ann Neurol 2009; 65:586.
25. VC Anderson et al. Pallidal vs subthalamic nucleus deep brain stimulation in Parkinson disease. Arch Neurol 2005; 62:554.
26. G Kleiner-Fishman et al. Subthalamic nucleus deep brain stimulation: summary and meta-analysis of outcomes. Mov Disord 2006; 21:S290.

Drugs for Parkinson's Disease

27. M Schüpbach et al. Neurosurgery in Parkinson disease: a distressed mind in a repaired body? Neurology 2006; 66:1811.
28. HM Smeding et al. Neuropsychological effects of bilateral STN stimulation in Parkinson disease: a controlled study. Neurology 2006; 66:1830.
29. M Menza et al. A controlled trial of antidepressants in patients with Parkinson disease and depression. Neurology 2009; 72:886.
30. JM Miyasaki et al. Practice parameter: evaluation and treatment of depression, psychosis, and dementia in Parkinson disease (an evidence-based review): report of the Quality Standards Subcommittee of the American Academy of Neurology. Neurology 2006; 66:996.
31. M Emre et al. Rivastigmine for dementia associated with Parkinson's disease. N Engl J Med 2004; 351:2509.
32. Memantine for Alzheimer's disease. Med Lett Drugs Ther 2003; 45:73.

DRUGS FOR
Peptic Ulcer Disease and GERD

Original publication date – September 2011 (revised March 2012)

RECOMMENDATIONS: All patients with peptic ulcer disease (PUD) need treatment with antisecretory drugs; proton pump inhibitors (PPIs) are more effective than H2-receptor antagonists (H2RAs). Omeprazole generally is as effective as any other PPI; it is available generically and over the counter (OTC). All H2RAs are available generically and OTC. When patients with peptic ulcer disease are infected with *Helicobacter pylori*, eradication of the infection with a combination of antibacterial drugs markedly decreases the incidence of recurrence.

Medical therapy for gastroesophageal reflux disease (GERD) is usually based on acid suppression. Antacid and H2RA therapy may be adequate for patients with mild, intermittent symptoms. Treatment with a PPI is preferred for more severe disease.

Peptic ulcer disease (PUD) is usually caused by non-steroidal anti-inflammatory drugs (NSAIDs) or by infection with *Helicobacter pylori*. Gastroesophageal reflux disease (GERD) can be caused by transient lower esophageal sphincter relaxation, reduced lower esophageal sphincter tone, hiatal hernia, delayed gastric emptying or hormonal changes due to pregnancy. Acid suppressive therapy is the cornerstone of management for both PUD and GERD.

DRUGS

H2-RECEPTOR ANTAGONISTS (H2RAs) — Currently available H2RAs are listed in the table that begins on page 246. These drugs inhibit the action of histamine at the H2-receptor of the parietal cell, decreasing basal acid secretion and, to a lesser degree, food-stimulated acid secretion. All of the H2RAs are about equally effective for treatment of PUD and GERD. They are not as effective as proton pump inhibitors (PPIs).

Adverse Effects – Severe adverse effects are uncommon with H2RAs, but headache, lethargy, confusion, depression and hallucinations can occur. Rarely, these agents have been associated with hepatitis and hematologic toxicity. Cimetidine is weakly anti-androgenic and may rarely cause reversible impotence and gynecomastia with chronic use.

Drug Interactions – Cimetidine moderately inhibits the activity of hepatic enzymes CYP1A2, 2C19, 2D6 and 3A4. Clinically significant adverse effects have occurred when cimetidine was used with drugs that are both metabolized by these enzymes and have a narrow therapeutic window, such as theophylline (*Theo-Dur*, and others), warfarin (*Coumadin*, and others), phenytoin (*Dilantin*, and others) or lidocaine (*Xylocaine*, and others). Ranitidine, famotidine and nizatidine are much less likely to interfere with the hepatic metabolism of other drugs.

Tolerance and Rebound – Repeated administration of H2RAs leads to pharmacologic tolerance and decreased effectiveness over time and has been associated with development of new dyspeptic symptoms.[1,2] While the mechanism is unclear, tolerance seems to be more prevalent in patients who are not infected with *H. pylori*.[3] Rebound acid hypersecretion can occur following discontinuation of H2RAs.

PROTON PUMP INHIBITORS (PPIs) — Currently available PPIs are also listed in the table. These drugs bind to the activated proton pump of the parietal cell, inhibiting secretion of hydrogen ions into the gastric lumen.

PPIs heal peptic ulcers more rapidly than H2RAs. Standard doses inhibit more than 90% of 24-hour acid secretion, compared to 50-80% with H2RAs. PPIs have short serum half-lives, but their duration of action is longer, allowing for once-daily dosing in most patients. Unlike H2RAs, tolerance does not occur with PPIs. Rebound dyspeptic symptoms and acid hypersecretion have been reported following discontinuation of a PPI.[4]

Adverse Effects – PPIs are generally well tolerated. Headache, nausea, abdominal pain, constipation, flatulence and diarrhea can occur. Gynecomastia and hepatic failure have occurred rarely. Subacute myopathy, arthralgia, severe rash, acute interstitial nephritis and hypomagnesemia have been reported.[5,6]

Acid suppression may increase the risk of bacterial gastroenteritis and *Clostridium difficile*-associated colitis. Long-term use of PPIs, particularly at high doses, has been associated with an increased risk of fractures in patients with osteoporosis and in other high-risk groups[7,8]; a cause and effect relationship has not been established, and PPI treatment has not been associated with osteoporosis.[9] Decreased absorption and subsequent deficiency of vitamin B_{12} can occur with chronic use of PPIs and/or H2RAs, particularly in elderly patients.

Drug Interactions – All PPIs may decrease serum concentrations of drugs that require gastric acidity for absorption, such as itraconazole (*Sporanox*, and others). The PPIs omeprazole and esomeprazole strongly inhibit the activity of the hepatic enzyme CYP2C19, possibly decreasing the metabolism of diazepam (*Valium*, and others), phenytoin (*Dilantin*, and others) and other drugs. Clopidogrel *(Plavix)* is converted to its active form by CYP2C19; inhibition of CYP2C19 may interfere with activation of clopidogrel and diminish its antiplatelet effect. The FDA warns against use of omeprazole with clopidogrel, but some studies have suggested that such use does not lead to an increase in adverse cardiovascular outcomes.[10,11] Still, if a patient taking clopidogrel needs a PPI, an alternative PPI, such as pantoprazole, could be considered.[12]

SUCRALFATE — An aluminum hydroxide complex of sucrose said to protect the ulcer from exposure to acid, sucralfate (*Carafate*, and others) has been used for acute treatment and prevention of recurrent peptic ulcers. Multiple daily doses are required, and it may not be effective in relieving ulcer pain.

Adverse Effects – Sucralfate is generally well tolerated, but may cause constipation and aluminum toxicity.

Drug Interactions – Sucralfate decreases absorption of some drugs; it should be taken at least two hours after ketoconazole (*Nizoral*, and others) and fluoroquinolones.

MISOPROSTOL — Misoprostol (*Cytotec*, and others), a prostaglandin E1 analog, can prevent gastric and duodenal ulcers in patients on chronic NSAID therapy. It may be as effective as a PPI in preventing NSAID-related ulcers, but requires multiple daily doses and is not as well tolerated. It has no established role in healing ulcers.

Adverse Effects – Abdominal pain and dose-related diarrhea are the most common adverse effects of misoprostol. Severe nausea can also occur. Misoprostol is an abortifacient and should not be used in women who could become pregnant.

ANTACIDS — Aluminum- and magnesium-containing antacids can be helpful in transiently relieving the symptoms of PUD and GERD. Aluminum-based antacids can be constipating, and magnesium-based antacids can cause diarrhea. Antacids may decrease absorption of some other drugs.

PEPTIC ULCER DISEASE

The first step in the management of PUD is to identify potential underlying causes such as NSAID use or *H. pylori* infection. Eradication of *H.*

pylori can promote healing and prevent recurrences of both duodenal and gastric ulcers.[13]

TESTING FOR *H. PYLORI* — The sensitivity of urea-based tests (breath and biopsy) and the stool antigen test for *H. pylori* is reduced by use of PPIs, bismuth or antibiotics. Patients should not take these drugs for at least 2 weeks before testing.

Urea breath tests *(BreathTek*; *PYtest)* can be used for office-based diagnosis. The patient ingests a urea solution or capsule labeled with a carbon isotope and then breathes into a container; in the presence of *H. pylori*, urease hydrolyzes the urea to release labeled CO_2, which can be detected by a mass spectrometer. These tests typically have >90% sensitivity and specificity.[14] The *BreathTek*, used with a desktop infrared spectrometer, can provide results within a few minutes.

Stool Antigens – A stool antigen enzyme immunoassay *(Premier Platinum HpSA)* has a sensitivity of about 94% and specificity of about 90%.[15] While it is reliable in confirming successful treatment, the stool antigen test should not be used to test for eradication of *H. pylori* until at least 4 weeks after completion of therapy.

Serology – Serologic antibody tests for *H. pylori* are useful in ruling out the diagnosis, but they lack specificity and are not reliable (because of persisting antibodies) for documenting eradication.

Biopsy – Endoscopic biopsy of the gastric mucosa permits identification of *H. pylori* by detection of its urease activity, by histology or by culture. Histology is the diagnostic gold standard for *H. pylori* detection. Urease testing of biopsy specimens can provide a rapid diagnosis. Culture is used mainly for antibiotic sensitivity testing to detect resistant organisms.

TREATMENT OF *H. PYLORI* — Regimens for treatment of *H. pylori* are listed in the table on page 250. In large clinical trials, combinations of

Drugs for Peptic Ulcer Disease and GERD

SOME DRUGS FOR PEPTIC ULCER DISEASE/GERD

Drug	Usual Dosage[1]
H2-RECEPTOR ANTAGONISTS[2]	
Cimetidine – generic	200-400 mg bid
Tagamet (GlaxoSmithKline)	
Tagamet HB (OTC) generic	
Famotidine[3] – generic	10-20 mg bid
Pepcid (Merck)	
Pepcid AC (OTC)	
generic	
Pepcid Complete (OTC)[4]	1 tab once daily
Nizatidine – generic	75-150 mg bid
Axid (Lilly)	
Axid AR (OTC)	
Ranitidine – generic	75-150 mg bid
Zantac (GlaxoSmithKline)	
Zantac (OTC)	
generic	
PROTON PUMP INHIBITORS[5]	
Dexlansoprazole – *Dexilant* (Takeda)	30-60 mg once daily
Esomeprazole[6] – *Nexium* (AstraZeneca)	20-40 mg once daily
Lansoprazole – generic	15-30 mg once daily
Prevacid (Takeda)	
Prevacid 24 HR (OTC)	
Omeprazole – generic	20-40 mg once daily
Prilosec (AstraZeneca)	
Prilosec OTC	
generic	
Zegerid	
Zegerid OTC	
Pantoprazole – generic	20-40 mg once daily
Protonix (Pfizer)	
Rabeprazole – *Aciphex* (Janssen)	20 mg once daily

OTC = Over the counter; ODT = orally disintegrating tabs.
1. The lower end of the range is generally used for initial treatment of GERD. Higher doses may be used in patients with peptic ulcers, hypersecretory states like Zollinger-Ellison Syndrome or for treatment of *H. pylori*.
2. Taking the total daily dose at once in the evening can also be effective.
3. Also available in combination with ibuprofen *(Duexis)*.

246

Some Available Formulations

200, 300, 400, 800 mg tabs; 300 mg/2mL soln for inj; 300 mg/5mL oral soln

200 mg tabs
20, 40 mg tabs; 10 mg/mL soln for inj; 40 mg/5mL susp

10, 20 mg tabs; 20 mg chewable tabs

10 mg chewable tabs
150, 300 mg caps; 15 mg/mL oral soln

75 mg tabs
150, 300 mg tabs, caps; 25 mg/mL soln for inj; 15 mg/mL oral syrup
150, 300 mg tabs; 25 mg/mL soln for inj; 15 mg/mL oral syrup
75, 150 mg tabs

30, 60 mg caps
20, 40 mg caps; 10, 20, 40 mg powder for susp; 20, 40 mg vial for inj
15, 30 mg ODT; 15, 30 mg caps

15 mg caps
10, 20, 40 mg caps
10, 20, 40 mg caps; 2.5, 10 mg granules for susp
20 mg tabs

20, 40 mg caps[7]; 20, 40 mg powder for susp
20 mg caps[7]
20, 40 mg tabs
20, 40 mg tabs; 40 mg granules for susp; 40 mg powder for inj
20 mg tabs

4. Also contains calcium carbonate 800 mg and magnesium hydroxide 165 mg.
5. PPIs are generally taken 30-60 minutes before the first meal of the day. Taking one before the evening meal may be more effective for nocturnal acid control.
6. Also available in combination with naproxen *(Vimovo)*.
7. Each capsule contains sodium bicarbonate 1.1 g; therefore, two 20-mg caps are not equivalent to a 40-mg cap.

Continued on next page.

Drugs for Peptic Ulcer Disease and GERD

SOME DRUGS FOR PEPTIC ULCER DISEASE/GERD (continued)

Drug	Usual Dosage[1]
OTHER DRUGS	
Misoprostol[8,9] – generic	200 mcg bid-tid
Cytotec (Searle)	
Sucralfate – generic	1 g qid
Carafate (Aventis)	

8. FDA-approved only for prevention of NSAID-associated gastric ulcers.

antimicrobial drugs active against *H. pylori* have been successful in eradicating the organism in up to 90% of patients. In practice, eradication rates are considerably lower due to increasing resistance to clarithromycin and metronidazole and poor patient adherence to these multi-drug regimens.

Eradication rates with commonly prescribed triple therapy regimens have fallen below 80%. Quadruple therapy and sequential therapy have higher rates of eradication. A recent study found no difference between sequential therapy and quadruple therapy, with both achieving eradication rates of 92-93%.[16] Quadruple therapy should be considered for initial treatment in areas with a high rate (>20%) of clarithromycin-resistant *H. pylori*.[17,18]

Patients should be tested for successful eradication of *H. pylori* and those still infected after treatment with 2 different regimens should receive salvage therapy with a different regimen, such as a PPI, amoxicillin and levofloxacin (*Levaquin*, and others), if needed.[13]

Adverse Effects – Bismuth subsalicylate temporarily turns the tongue and stool black and can cause tinnitus. Amoxicillin may cause diarrhea.

248

Some Available Formulations

100, 200 mcg tabs

1 g tabs; 1 g/10 mL oral susp

9. Also available in combination with diclofenac *(Arthrotec)*.

Metronidazole, tinidazole and tetracycline frequently cause mild gastrointestinal disturbances, and metronidazole causes a metallic taste. Clarithromycin causes fewer gastrointestinal symptoms, but commonly causes disturbances in taste that some patients find intolerable. Clarithromycin, metronidazole and tetracycline can all interact adversely with many other drugs. Both metronidazole and tinidazole can cause a disulfiram-type reaction to alcohol.

GASTROESOPHAGEAL REFLUX DISEASE

GERD is typically a benign condition, although complications such as strictures and Barrett's esophagus can occur, and the risk of esophageal adenocarcinoma is increased. Patients <55 years old presenting with typical, uncomplicated GERD can be treated empirically with lifestyle modification and acid-suppressive therapy. Patients ≥55 years old presenting with heartburn or dyspepsia should have an endoscopy.[19]

LIFESTYLE MODIFICATION — Common maneuvers include avoiding recumbancy for at least 3 hours after a meal and elevating the head of the bed. Foods and drugs that decrease lower esophageal sphincter pressure (chocolate, alcohol, peppermint, coffee, tobacco and

Drugs for Peptic Ulcer Disease and GERD

SOME MULTI-DRUG REGIMENS FOR *HELICOBACTER PYLORI*

Drug	Daily Dose	Duration[1]
TRIPLE THERAPY		
Clarithromycin (*Biaxin,* and others)	500 mg bid	10-14 days
+ Amoxicillin (*Amoxil,* and others)	1 g bid	
or Metronidazole[2] (*Flagyl,* and others)	500 mg bid	
+ a PPI[3]		
QUADRUPLE THERAPY		
Bismuth subsalicylate (*PeptoBismol,* and others)	2 tablets (525 mg) tid or qid or 30 mL tid or qid	14 days
+ Metronidazole (*Flagyl,* and others)	500 mg tid or qid	
+ Tetracycline (*Sumycin,* and others)	500 mg tid or qid	
+ a PPI[3] or H2RA		
SEQUENTIAL THERAPY		
+ Amoxicillin (*Amoxil,* and others) a PPI[3]	1 g bid	5 days
followed by:		
+ Clarithromycin (*Biaxin,* and others)	500 mg bid	5 days
+ Tinidazole *(Tindamax)* a PPI[3]	500 mg bid	
COMBINATION PRODUCTS		
Helidac Therapy	14 daily blister cards, each containing 8 bismuth subsalicylate 262.4-mg chewable tabs, 4 metronidazole 250-mg tabs and 4 tetracycline 500-mg caps	
Prevpac	14 daily blister cards, each containing 2 lansoprazole 30-mg caps, 4 amoxicillin 500-mg caps and 2 clarithromycin 500-mg tabs	
Pylera	120 capsules, each combining bismuth subcitrate potassium 140 mg, metronidazole 125 mg and tetracycline HCl 125 mg (3 caps qid)	

1. Antisecretory drugs may be needed longer to heal the ulcer.
2. For patients allergic to penicillin who have not previously received a macrolide or are unable to tolerate bismuth quadruple therapy.
3. Standard oral PPI dosages are: esomeprazole 40 mg once daily, lansoprazole 30 mg bid, omeprazole 20 mg bid, pantoprazole 40 mg bid, rabeprazole 20 mg bid.

carbonated beverages) and/or delay gastric emptying (fatty foods) are discouraged. For obese patients, weight loss may reduce the incidence of GERD symptoms.

ACID-SUPPRESSIVE THERAPY — Medications that suppress gastric acid are the mainstay of GERD therapy. Options include antacids, H2RAs and PPIs. The choice of drug depends on the severity and frequency of symptoms and the presence or absence of esophagitis.

Non-Erosive Reflux Disease (NERD) – Antacids and H2RAs may be adequate for symptom relief in patients with mild NERD. While these agents have similar peak potency, antacids have a faster onset of action and H2RAs have a longer duration of action (up to 10 hours).[20] PPIs are used less frequently for symptom relief because their onset of action is delayed. An immediate-release form of omeprazole *(Zegerid)* combines non-enteric-coated omeprazole with sodium bicarbonate.[21]

Patients with more severe NERD may require continuous therapy with an H2RA or a PPI. PPIs have been shown to maintain remission of symptoms and are generally preferred.[22]

Erosive Esophagitis – A PPI is the drug of choice for acute and chronic management of erosive esophagitis. PPIs decrease symptoms and heal esophagitis more effectively than other drugs. In one study, symptom relief occurred in 27% of patients treated with placebo, in 60% with an H2RA and in 83% with a PPI, and healing of esophageal erosions occurred in 24% of patients treated with placebo, in 50% treated with an H2RA and in 78% treated with a PPI.[20]

ADJUNCTIVE TREATMENT — **Baclofen** (*Lioresal*, and others) is a gamma-aminobutyric acid (B) ($GABA_B$) receptor agonist that inhibits transient lower esophageal sphincter relaxation and decreases postprandial acid reflux in patients with GERD.[23] It is effective in reducing symptoms among patients refractory to PPI therapy.[24] Baclofen is not approved by the FDA for use in GERD. Common side effects include drowsiness, dizziness, lightheadedness, hypotension and nausea.

GERD IN PREGNANCY — Heartburn occurs in approximately 30-50% of pregnancies, and is largely attributed to a progesterone-mediated decrease in lower esophageal sphincter tone. Antacids can be helpful, but those containing sodium bicarbonate should be avoided during pregnancy due to the risks of maternal or fetal alkalosis and fluid overload.[25] H2RAs are classified as category B (no evidence of risk in humans) for use during pregnancy. Although generally considered safe, clinical data on the use of PPIs during pregnancy are limited. A meta-analysis evaluating first-trimester use (predominantly of omeprazole) found no increased risk of congenital malformations and a recent cohort study confirmed these findings.[26,27] PPIs are classified as pregnancy category B, with the exception of omeprazole, which is category C (risk cannot be ruled out).

SURGERY — Weight loss surgery has variable effects on GERD: Roux-en-Y gastric bypass is associated with a decrease in GERD and dyspeptic symptoms, but gastric banding and gastric sleeve have not consistently shown the same benefit.[28]

Laparoscopic fundoplication is the primary surgical procedure for management of GERD; the gastric fundus is wrapped around the gastroesophageal junction either partially or completely, creating a mechanical barrier.[29] It has not been shown to be superior to medical therapy. At least one third of patients treated with fundoplication will still require chronic acid-suppressive therapy for ongoing reflux symptoms. Dysphagia is common in the early post-operative period and may require early endoscopic dilation, but typically resolves after 2-3 months. In some patients, dysphagia persists and may require endoscopic dilation or surgical revision. Postprandial bloating (gas-bloat syndrome), increased flatus and diarrhea are common postoperatively.

ENDOSCOPIC THERAPY — Various modalities of endoscopic reflux therapy have been tried, including application of radiofrequency energy to the gastroesophageal junction, suture plication of the proximal stomach, and either injection of a biopolymer or implantation of a bioprosthesis at the level of the lower esophageal sphincter. Convincing data supporting use of these techniques are lacking, and none are approved by the FDA.[30,31]

1. L Lachman and CW Howden. Twenty-four hour intragastric pH: tolerance within 5 days of continuous ranitidine administration. Am J Gastroenterol 2000; 95:57.
2. K Furuta et al. Tolerance to H2 receptor antagonist correlates well with the decline in efficacy against gastroesophageal reflux in patients with gastroesophageal reflux disease. J Gastroenterol Hepatol 2006; 21:1581.
3. T Fujisawa et al. Helicobacter pylori infection prevents the occurrence of the tolerance phenomenon of histamine H2 receptor antagonists. Aliment Pharmacol Ther 2004; 20:559.
4. A Niklasson et al. Dyspeptic symptom development after discontinuation of a proton pump inhibitor: a double-blind placebo-controlled trial. Am J Gastroenterol 2010; 105:1531.
5. In brief: PPIs and hypomagnesemia. Med Lett Drugs Ther 2011; 53:25.
6. TW Furlanetto and GA Faulhaber. Hypomagnesemia and proton pump inhibitors: below the tip of the iceberg. Arch Intern Med 2011; 171:1391.
7. EW Yu et al. Proton pump inhibitors and risk of fractures: a meta-analysis of 11 international studies. Am J Med 2011; 124:519.
8. S Ngamruengphong et al. Proton pump inhibitors and risk of fracture: a systematic review and meta-analysis of observational studies. Am J Gastroenterol 2011; 106:1209.
9. LE Targownik et al. Proton pump inhibitor use is not associated with osteoporosis or accelerated bone mineral density loss. Gastroenterology 2010; 138:896.
10. DL Bhatt et al. Clopidogrel with or without omeprazole in coronary artery disease. N Engl J Med 2010; 363:1909.
11. KJ Harjai et al. Clinical outcomes in patients with the concomitant use of clopidogrel and proton pump inhibitors after percutaneous coronary intervention: an analysis from the Guthrie Health Off-Label Stent (GHOST) investigators. Circ Cardiovasc Interv 2011; 4:162.
12. In brief: clopidogrel and omeprazole. Med Lett Drugs Ther 2010; 52:93.
13. WD Chey and BC Wong. American College of Gastroenterology guideline on the management of Helicobacter pylori infection. Am J Gastroenterol 2007; 102:1808.
14. RJ Saad and WD Chey. Breath tests for gastrointestinal disease: the real deal or just a lot of hot air? Gastroenterology 2007; 133:1763.
15. L Gatta et al. Non-invasive techniques for the diagnosis of Helicobacter pylori infection. Clin Microbiol Infect 2003; 9:489.

Drugs for Peptic Ulcer Disease and GERD

16. DY Graham and L Fischbach. Helicobacter pylori treatment in the era of increasing antibiotic resistance. Gut 2010; 59:1143.
17. KE McColl. Clinical Practice. Helicobacter pylori infection. N Engl J Med 2011; 362:1599.
18. E Rimbara et al. Optimal therapy for Helicobacter pylori infections. Nat Rev Gastroenterol Hepatol 2011; 8:79.
19. NJ Talley et al. Guidelines for the management of dyspepsia. Am J Gastroenterol 2005; 100:2324.
20. KR DeVault and DO Castell. Updated guidelines for the diagnosis and treatment of gastroesophageal reflux disease. Am J Gastroenterol 2005; 100:190.
21. Zegerid – immediate-release omeprazole. Med Lett Drugs Ther 2005; 47:29.
22. M Khan et al. Medical treatments in the short term management of reflux oesophagitis. Cochrane Database Syst Rev 2007 Apr 18; (2):CD003244.
23. Q Zhang et al. Control of transient lower oesophageal sphincter relaxations and reflux by the GABA(B) agonist baclofen in patients with gastro-oesophageal reflux disease. Gut 2002; 50:19.
24. GH Koek et al. Effect of the GABA(B) agonist baclofen in patients with symptoms and duodeno-gastro-oesophageal reflux refractory to proton pump inhibitors. Gut 2003; 52:1397.
25. JE Richter. Review article: the management of heartburn in pregnancy. Aliment Pharmacol Ther 2005; 22:749.
26. SK Gill et al. The safety of proton pump inhibitors (PPIs) in pregnancy: a meta-analysis. Am J Gastroenterol 2009; 104:1541.
27. B Pasternak and A Hviid. Use of proton pump inhibitors in early pregnancy and the rate of birth defects. N Engl J Med 2010; 363:2114.
28. R Tutuian. Obesity and GERD: pathophysiology and effect of bariatric surgery. Curr Gastroenterol Rep 2011; 13:205.
29. JP Galmiche et al. Laparoscopic antireflux surgery vs. esomeprazole treatment for chronic GERD: the LOTUS randomized clinical trial. JAMA 2011; 305:1969.
30. MP Schwartz and AJ Smout. Review article: the endoscopic treatment of gastro-oesophageal reflux disease. Aliment Pharmacol Ther 2007; 26 (Suppl 2):1.
31. H Louis and J Devière. Endoscopic-endoluminal therapies: a critical appraisal. Best Pract Res Clin Gastroenterol 2010; 24:969.

DRUGS FOR
Postmenopausal Osteoporosis

Original publication date – November 2011

RECOMMENDATIONS — Calcium supplements can decrease the risk of osteoporosis in patients with an inadequate intake of calcium and vitamin D. There is no evidence that patients with an adequate dietary intake of calcium and vitamin D will benefit from taking supplements.

Oral bisphosphonates can prevent vertebral and nonvertebral fractures in postmenopausal women with osteoporosis. Weekly or monthly doses of oral bisphosphonates are as effective as daily doses in increasing bone mineral density (BMD) and probably better tolerated, but fracture data are available only for once-daily formulations. IV administration of ibandronate every 3 months or zoledronic acid once a year is another alternative. The optimal duration of bisphosphonate therapy is unclear; available data, which are limited, indicate that some women continue to benefit from taking a bisphosphonate for as long as 10 years, and the benefit may outweigh the low risk of a bisphosphonate-induced atypical fracture.

Denosumab injected subcutaneously once every 6 months is the first non-bisphosphonate antiresorptive shown to reduce the risk of spine, hip and other nonvertebral fractures in women with postmenopausal osteoporosis; it may be an effective alternative in patients who have not responded to bisphosphonates or cannot tolerate them. Teriparatide, the 1-34 sequence of parathyroid hormone, offers another alternative; it improves bone density by increasing bone formation rather than by suppressing bone turnover.

Osteoporosis is characterized by low bone mass with microarchitectural disruption and skeletal fragility that results in an increased risk of fracture. The diagnosis has traditionally been established by bone densitometry, which is generally reported in terms of standard deviations (SD) from mean values in young adults (T-score). The World Health Organization (WHO) has defined normal bone mineral density (BMD) for women as a value within one SD of the young adult mean. Values 2.5 SD or more below the mean (T score -2.5) are defined as osteoporosis. The WHO has developed a computerized model (FRAX) that predicts the 10-year probability of a hip fracture or any other major osteoporotic fracture based on clinical risk factors and BMD at the femoral neck.[1]

CALCIUM AND VITAMIN D — Whether a lifelong increase in calcium intake decreases the risk of osteoporosis is unclear. Calcium supplementation can increase BMD in children and adolescents and reduce bone loss in postmenopausal women and older men,[2] but 3 randomized trials found that it did not reduce the fracture rate in older women.[3-5] A subgroup analysis of the largest of these trials, the Women's Health Initiative (WHI), reported a reduction in fractures among the women who were most adherent to calcium and vitamin D supplementation.[5] A meta-analysis in men and women ≥60 years old indicated that a minimum of 700 IU/d of vitamin D_3 (cholecalciferol), with or without calcium supplementation, could decrease the risk of nonvertebral fractures.[6] Another meta-analysis in men and women ≥50 years old reported that use of calcium alone or calcium plus vitamin D reduced fractures of all types, especially with calcium doses ≥1200 mg/d and with vitamin D ≥800 IU/d.[7]

Recommendations – The National Osteoporosis Foundation recommends dietary calcium as the preferred method to achieve adequate calcium intake and to use calcium supplements only if dietary intake is insufficient. The

SOME CALCIUM PRODUCTS

Drug	Ca^* (mg)	D_3^* (IU)	Tabs/d[1]
CALCIUM CARBONATE[2]			
Caltrate 600+D (Pfizer)	600	200	2
Os-Cal Extra+D_3 (GSK)	500	400	2
Tums E-X 750 (GSK)	300	—	4
Viactiv (McNeil)[3]	500	500	2
CALCIUM CITRATE[2]			
Citracal+D (Bayer)	315	250	2-4
Calcimate (GNC)	250	150	4
CALCIUM COMPLEX (CARBONATE, LACTATE, GLUCONATE)			
Calcet Plus (Mission)	250	200	4-6
CALCIUM PHOSPHATE			
Posture-D (Inverness)[4]	600	125	2

* Content per tablet.
1. Needed to provide about 1000 mg elemental calcium daily.
2. Available generically.
3. Available as a soft chewable preparation and in tablet form; also contains 40 mcg vitamin K.
4. Also contains 266 mg phosphorus.

Institute of Medicine (IOM) recommends a total daily elemental calcium intake of 1000 mg for all adults 19-50 years old, including pregnant and lactating women, 1000 mg for men 51-70 years old, and 1200 mg for women >50 years old and men >70 years old.[8] Calcium supplements are available in a variety of salts with varying concentrations of elemental calcium to compensate for deficiencies in dietary intake. Calcium citrate does not require acid for absorption, can be taken with or without food, and is preferred in patients taking proton pump inhibitors or H2-receptor antagonists or in those with achlorhydria. Calcium carbonate should be taken with food to enhance calcium absorption. Calcium supplementation of >500 mg/day should be given in divided doses to optimize absorption.

Vitamin D is necessary for optimal absorption of calcium. Exposure to sunlight leads to cutaneous synthesis of the vitamin. Vitamin D status can

Drugs for Postmenopausal Osteoporosis

CALCIUM CONTENT OF SOME FOODS[1]

Food	Serving size	Calcium content (mg)
Yogurt, lowfat, fruit-flavored	8 oz	345
Milk, skim	1 cup	299
Collards, cooked	1 cup	266
Swiss cheese	1 oz	219
Mozzarella cheese, part-skim	1 oz	207
Cheddar cheese	1 oz	204
Creamed cottage cheese	1 cup	174
Tofu, raw, firm	¼ block	163
Oatmeal, instant (fortified)	1 packet	142
Breakfast cereals, Cheerios[2]	1 cup	122
Mustard greens, cooked	1 cup	104
Kale, boiled	1 cup	94
Broccoli, boiled	1 cup	62
Figs, dried	2 figs	62
Parmesan cheese, grated	1 tbsp	55

1. US Department of Agriculture, National nutrient database for standard reference, release 24. http://www.ars.usda.gov/nutrientdata. Accessed October 3, 2011.
2. Calcium content varies, *Total Whole Grain* cereal (General Mills) contains 1000 mg of calcium per ¾ cup serving.

be evaluated by measuring serum concentrations of 25-hydroxy vitamin D (25-OH-D); a level of $\geq$20 ng/mL ($\geq$50 nmol/L) is considered acceptable. Some experts have suggested that levels $\geq$30 ng/mL may be desirable in older adults to help prevent fractures and falls.[9,10] The IOM recommends a dietary allowance of vitamin D of 600 IU daily for people up to 70 years old and 800 IU daily for those $\geq$71 years old.

Adverse Effects – Calcium supplements are generally well tolerated. Constipation, intestinal bloating and excess gas can occur. A slightly higher risk of kidney stones has been reported among women who take calcium supplements.[11] Some reports have suggested that calcium sup-

VITAMIN D CONTENT OF SOME FOODS[1]

Food	Serving size	Vitamin D content (IU)
Salmon, sockeye, cooked	3 oz	447
Halibut, cooked	3 oz	196
Sardines, canned	3 oz	164
Tuna, light canned	3 oz	154
Milk, whole (fortified)	8 oz	124
Milk, skim (fortified)	8 oz	115
Herring, pickled	3 oz	96
Egg, whole extra large	1	44

1. US Department of Agriculture, National nutrient database for standard reference, release 24. http://www.ars.usda.gov/nutrientdata. Accessed October 3, 2011. Breakfast cereals, margarine and many other products are often fortified with vitamin D.

plementation could increase the risk of cardiovascular disease, but in the Women's Health Initiative, among 36,000 postmenopausal women randomized to either calcium (1000 mg/day) plus vitamin D (400 IU/day) or placebo, 7 years of calcium plus vitamin D supplementation did not increase the incidence of myocardial infarction or stroke.[12] Two meta-analyses reported an increased risk of myocardial infarction in patients randomized to calcium with or without vitamin D supplements versus placebo.[13,14] A third meta-analysis did not show a significant increase in cardiovascular disease in patients supplementing with calcium, vitamin D or both.[15]

Hypercalciuria and hypercalcemia are manifestations of vitamin D toxicity. The IOM has defined the safe upper limit for vitamin D in adults as 4000 IU/day. Some reports have associated levels of 25-OH-D >40-50 ng/mL with an increased risk of fracture and possibly some cancers.[16-18]

BISPHOSPHONATES — These nonhormonal agents decrease bone resorption by binding to active sites of bone remodeling and inhibiting osteoclasts. Food, calcium supplements, antacids and other medications containing divalent cations, such as iron, may interfere with their absorption from the gastrointestinal (GI) tract. Fracture data for oral bisphosphonates are available only for once-daily formulations.

Alendronate – Alendronate (*Fosamax*, and others) is an oral bisphosphonate approved for daily or once-weekly use for prevention and treatment of osteoporosis. Weekly dosing appears to be as effective as daily dosing in increasing BMD and may be better tolerated. Alendronate is the only bisphosphonate available generically in the US that is FDA-approved for use in osteoporosis.

Among 1099 postmenopausal women who had received alendronate for 5 years and were randomized to an additional 5 years of alendronate or to placebo, those who received the additional years of alendronate had a significant decrease in clinically recognized vertebral fractures (2.4% vs. 5.3%), but not in nonvertebral fractures.[19] In a post hoc subset analysis of the same study, continuing alendronate for the full 10 years significantly reduced nonvertebral fracture risk in women with vertebral fractures whose femoral neck BMD T-scores were still -2.5 or worse after 5 years of alendronate treatment.[20] A study in 247 postmenopausal women with osteoporosis treated with alendronate for up to 10 years found that spinal BMD continued to increase throughout the study period; the lowest rate of clinical vertebral fractures occurred in women who took the drug for the entire 10-year period.[21]

Risedronate – The second oral bisphosphonate approved for prevention and treatment of osteoporosis in postmenopausal women, risedronate (*Actonel*) is available in daily, once-weekly and once-monthly formulations. An enteric-coated, delayed-release formulation (*Atelvia*) approved for treatment of postmenopausal osteoporosis is taken immediately after breakfast.[22] All of these formulations appear to have equivalent effects on BMD.[23,24]

A 3-year trial in about 1300 postmenopausal women (average age 69) with low bone mass and at least one vertebral fracture found 61 (11%) new vertebral fractures with daily risedronate and 93 (16%) with placebo, a significant difference. Nonvertebral fractures also decreased significantly in the group receiving risedronate compared to those receiving placebo (33 vs. 52). In an extension of this study, women were re-evaluated one year after discontinuing treatment. BMD decreased and bone turnover markers returned to baseline. The incidence of new vertebral fractures, however, remained significantly lower (6.5 vs. 11.6%) in the former risedronate users.[25]

Ibandronate – Oral ibandronate *(Boniva)* is approved for both prevention and treatment of postmenopausal osteoporosis. Daily oral ibandronate reduced the incidence of vertebral fractures in osteoporotic women, and appeared to reduce the incidence of nonvertebral fractures in a post hoc analysis of a small subgroup of high-risk women with markedly reduced femoral neck BMD.[26] Monthly oral ibandronate appears to be at least as effective as daily dosing in increasing BMD and at least as well tolerated as taking the drug daily.

Intravenous (IV) ibandronate has also been approved for the treatment of postmenopausal osteoporosis. In a non-inferiority trial, 1395 postmenopausal women with osteoporosis were randomized to ibandronate 3 mg IV every 3 months, 2 mg IV every 2 months, or 2.5 mg oral ibandronate daily. After 2 years, the increase in lumbar spine BMD, the primary endpoint, was significantly greater with the IV regimens: 6.3% with the 3 mg IV dose, 6.4% with 2 mg and 4.8% with the oral dose.[27] Two meta-analyses have found a reduction in nonvertebral fractures with high-dose oral or IV ibandronate, but no direct fracture protection data are available specifically for IV ibandronate.[28,29]

Zoledronic Acid – Zoledronic acid *(Reclast)* is the first bisphosphonate approved by the FDA for once-yearly IV treatment of osteoporosis in

Drugs for Postmenopausal Osteoporosis

SOME DRUGS FOR OSTEOPOROSIS

Drug	FDA-Approved Indication
ORAL BISPHOSPHONATES[2]	
Alendronate – generic	Prevention
Fosamax (Merck)[3]	Treatment
Fosamax Plus D	Treatment
Ibandronate – *Boniva* (Roche)	Prevention, Treatment
Risedronate – *Actonel* (Warner Chilcott)	Prevention, Treatment
delayed-release	
Atelvia (Warner Chilcott)	Treatment
INTRAVENOUS (IV) BISPHOSPHONATES	
Ibandronate –	
Boniva (Roche)	Treatment
Zoledronic acid[4] –	
Reclast (Novartis)	Treatment
	Prevention
SELECTIVE ESTROGEN RECEPTOR MODULATOR	
Raloxifene – *Evista* (Lilly)	Prevention, Treatment
ANTI-RANK LIGAND ANTIBODY	
Denosumab – *Prolia* (Amgen)[5]	Treatment
CALCITONIN	
Fortical Nasal Spray (Upsher-Smith)	Treatment
Miacalcin Nasal Spray (Novartis)	Treatment
Miacalcin Injection (Novartis)	Treatment
PARATHYROID HORMONE	
Teriparatide – *Forteo* (Lilly)	Treatment

1. In patients with normal renal function
2. Alendronate, ibandronate and risedronate are also available as smaller tablets for daily use.
3. *Fosamax* is also available in a 70 mg/75 mL liquid formulation.
4. Zoledronic acid is also available in a 4-mg formulation *(Zometa)* for treatment of hypercalcemia of malignancy, multiple myeloma and bone metastases from solid tumors.

Dosage[1]

35 mg/wk
70 mg/wk
70 mg + 2800 IU D_3/wk
70 mg + 5600 IU D_3/wk
150 mg/mo
35 mg/wk
150 mg/mo

35 mg/wk

3 mg IV once every 3 months

5 mg IV once/yr
5 mg IV once every 2 years

60 mg/d

60 mg SC every 6 months

200 IU (1 spray) intranasal/d
200 IU (1 spray) intranasal/d
100 IU SC or IM every other day

20 mcg SC/d

5. Denosumab is also available in a 120 mg/1.7mL formulation *(Xgeva)* for prevention of skeletal-related events in patients with bone metastases from solid tumors.

postmenopausal women.[30] In the 3-year HORIZON Pivotal Fracture Trial, new hip fractures occurred in 52 of 3875 women (1.4%) infused annually with 5 mg of IV zoledronic acid vs. 88 of 3861 (2.5%) infused with placebo, a significant difference. Other nonvertebral fractures and clinical vertebral fractures were also significantly decreased in drug-treated patients.[31] The duration of action, the optimal duration of treatment and its long-term safety (>3 years) have not been established. Studies in osteopenic postmenopausal women suggest that a single 5-mg IV dose of zoledronic acid can suppress bone turnover and increase BMD for up to 3 years.[32]

Adverse Effects – Oral alendronate, risedronate and ibandronate can cause heartburn, esophageal irritation, esophagitis, abdominal pain, diarrhea and other adverse GI effects. To ensure adequate absorption and prevent esophageal injury, they must be taken after an overnight fast, while in an upright position, along with 8 ounces of plain (not mineral) water. After taking the drug, the patient must take nothing by mouth except plain water for at least 30 minutes (60 minutes with ibandronate) and avoid lying down. GI adverse effects have occurred even when patients followed these instructions. The enteric-coated, delayed-release once-weekly formulation of risedronate *(Atelvia)* is taken immediately after breakfast with at least 4 ounces of water and then the patient must remain upright for at least 30 minutes; diarrhea and abdominal pain occurred more often with this formulation than with risedronate 5 mg daily (8.8% vs. 4.9% and 5.2% vs. 2.9%, respectively).

The FDA has received reports of 23 patients in the US and 31 in Europe and Japan diagnosed as having esophageal cancer while taking oral bisphosphonates.[33] Mean latency from bisphosphonate use to cancer diagnosis was ≥3 years in the US and 2 years in Europe and Japan. A study examining data from European national registries did not show an increased risk of esophageal cancer in patients who had filled more than one prescription for any oral bisphosphonate during a mean follow-up period of 2.8 years and a mean duration of exposure to oral bisphosphonates of 2.1 years.[34] In one case-cohort study, >41,000 patients who used bisphosphonates were compared to a similar number of controls matched for age and gender over a mean follow-up period of about 4.5 years; this study found no increase in the risk of esophageal cancer in the bisphosphonate group.[35]

Severe bone, joint and muscle pain have occurred with the bisphosphonates.[36] Ocular inflammation has also been reported. Hypocalcemia can occur, typically in those with vitamin D deficiency. IV bisphosphonates have been associated with an acute phase reaction (low-grade fevers, myalgias and arthralgias) within 1-3 days of the infusion, most frequently after the first infusion; NSAIDs or acetaminophen can decrease these symptoms. Acute phase reactions have also been reported with monthly formulations of oral bisphosphonates. Osteonecrosis of the jaw (ONJ) has been described with chronic use of bisphosphonates.[37] The majority of cases have occurred in cancer patients or in immunocompromised patients given IV bisphosphonates. A weak association has been reported between bisphosphonate use and an increased incidence of atrial arrhythmias.[38]

The FDA has reported cases of renal failure requiring dialysis and deaths in patients with decreased renal function treated with zoledronic acid.[39]

Long-term Bone Strength – Alendronate may remain in bone for as long as 10 years. Whether long-term suppression of bone turnover could weaken bone rather than strengthen it is unknown. Case reports have described atypical low-energy fractures of the femoral shaft in patients on long-term bisphosphonates.[40] In a nested case-control study of 205,466 women ≥68 years old, treatment with a bisphosphonate for ≥5 years was associated with a higher incidence of subtrochanteric or femoral shaft fracture (adjusted OR 2.74, 95% CI 1.25-6.02) and a lower incidence of typical (femoral neck and intertrochanteric) osteoporotic fractures (OR 0.76, 95% CI 0.63-0.93) as compared to transient use (<100 days). Using a bisphosphonate for <5 years was not associated with a significant increase in subtrochanteric or femoral shaft fracture risk. Among the >52,000 women with at least 5 years of bisphosphonate use, the estimated absolute risk of having a subtrochanteric or femoral shaft fracture during the subsequent year was 0.13% and within 2 years was 0.22%.[41] Some clinicians stop bisphosphonates after 5 years in patients at low risk of fracture (stable bone density, no history of fractures) and resume the drug if bone turnover markers increase or BMD falls. Overall, there is no consensus on the optimal duration of bisphosphonate treatment.

RALOXIFENE — Raloxifene *(Evista)*[42] is a selective estrogen receptor modulator (SERM) with estrogen-like effects on bone and antiestrogen effects on the uterus and breast. Approved by the FDA for both prevention and treatment of postmenopausal osteoporosis, it has reduced the risk of vertebral fractures, but not nonvertebral fractures.[43]

Adverse Effects – Hot flashes, leg cramps and peripheral edema can occur in patients taking raloxifene. Like estrogens, raloxifene increases the risk of thromboembolic events, including fatal stroke.

ESTROGEN — In some women, lack of estrogen after menopause is associated with rapid bone loss. A number of estrogen products (see Table) are available for prevention of osteoporosis, but given its adverse effect profile, estrogen is no longer used as a first-line therapy for prevention of postmenopausal osteoporosis.

Adverse Effects – Estrogen plus a progestin has been associated with an increased incidence of coronary events (cardiac death or myocardial infarction), stroke, pulmonary emboli and breast cancer. Long-term use of estrogen may also increase the risk of ovarian cancer.

PARATHYROID HORMONE — Unlike other drugs available for osteoporosis, which act by decreasing bone turnover, low-dose intermittent subcutaneous injection of parathyroid hormone (PTH) increases bone density by stimulating bone formation. Teriparatide *(Forteo)*, the 1-34 sequence of PTH, was approved by the FDA for treatment of osteoporosis for up to 2 years (in the patient's lifetime) in both men and postmenopausal women at high risk for fractures.

Injections of teriparatide once daily have been shown to increase BMD and to decrease the incidence of vertebral and nonvertebral fractures by 50% or more; retreatment after a drug-free period has been shown to produce further gains in BMD.[44,45]

Adverse Effects – Adverse effects of PTH have included nausea, headache, dizziness and muscle cramps. Hypercalcemia has been reported; it can generally be corrected by decreasing calcium or vitamin D supplementation. The FDA, based on animal data, has included a boxed warning in the labeling regarding a risk of osteosarcoma.

CALCITONIN — Salmon calcitonin, a peptide hormone given intranasally, subcutaneously or intramuscularly, is approved by the FDA for treatment of osteoporosis. It decreases bone resorption by inhibiting osteoclast function. It may also have an analgesic effect. A 5-year trial in 1200 women with osteoporosis found new vertebral fractures in 51 of 287 (18%) receiving a 200 IU dose of calcitonin nasal spray once daily and in 70 of 270 (26%) receiving a placebo, a statistically significant difference. The incidence of vertebral fractures with a higher dose of 400 IU (61/278; 22%) was not significantly lower than with placebo.[46]

Adverse Effects – Rhinitis and occasional epistaxis have occurred with intranasal calcitonin. Nausea and flushing can occur with the parenteral formulations. Serious allergic reactions including anaphylaxis have been reported.

DENOSUMAB — Denosumab *(Prolia)* is a fully human monoclonal antibody against RANK ligand that inhibits osteoclast formation and reduces bone resorption. Injected subcutaneously every 6 months, it has been shown to increase BMD and reduce the incidence of new vertebral,

Drugs for Postmenopausal Osteoporosis

SOME ESTROGEN PREPARATIONS FOR OSTEOPOROSIS

Estrogen Preparations[1]	FDA-Approved Indication
ORAL ESTROGENS Estradiol, micronized – generic 　*Estrace* (Warner Chilcott) Esterified estrogens – *Menest* (Pfizer) Estropipate – generic 　*Ortho-est* (Women FH) Conjugated equine estrogens 　*Premarin* (Pfizer)	Prevention
ORAL ESTROGEN-PROGESTIN COMBINATIONS Estradiol/norgestimate 　*Prefest* (Teva) Estradiol/norethindrone acetate 　*Activella* (Novo Nordisk) 　*Femhrt* (Warner Chilcott) Conjugated equine estrogens/medroxyprogesterone 　*Premphase* (Pfizer) 　*Prempro* (Pfizer)	Prevention
TRANSDERMAL ESTROGENS Estradiol, transdermal 　generic 　*Alora* (Watson) 　*Climara* (Bayer) 　*Estraderm* (Novartis) 　*Menostar* (Bayer) 　*Vivelle* (Novartis) 　*Vivelle-Dot*	Prevention
TRANSDERMAL ESTROGEN-PROGESTIN COMBINATION Estradiol/levonorgestrel, transdermal 　*Climara Pro* (Bayer)	Prevention

1. Estrogen products are available in many sizes. For a woman with an intact uterus, a progestin must be added to estrogen therapy. Oral estrogens are usually given continuously or in a cyclic regimen.

Dosage

0.5 mg/d

0.3 mg/d
0.75 mg/d

0.3 mg/d

1 mg/d x 3 days, alternate
  with 1 mg/0.9 mg x3d

0.5 mg/0.1 mg-1 mg/0.5 mg/d
5 mg/1 mg/d

0.625 mg/d on days 1-14, then
0.625 mg/5 mg/d on days 15-28
0.3 mg/1.5 mg/d

15.5 cm^2 patch/wk (0.05 mg/d)
18 cm^2 patch 2x/wk (0.05 mg/d)
6.5 cm^2 patch/wk (0.025 mg/d)
10 cm^2 patch 2x/wk (0.05 mg/d)
3.25 cm^2 patch once/wk (0.014 mg/d)
7.25 cm^2 patch 2x/wk (0.025 mg/d)
2.5 cm^2 patch 2x/wk (0.025 mg/d)

22 cm^2 patch/wk (0.45 mg/0.015 mg/d)

hip and other nonvertebral fractures in postmenopausal women.[47] No studies are available directly comparing the efficacy of denosumab and bisphosphonates in preventing fractures.

Denosumab's effects on BMD and bone turnover are reversible with discontinuation of the drug. After a 24-month course of denosumab, increases in bone turnover occurred 3 months after the drug was discontinued and declines in BMD to pre-treatment values occurred at 1 and 2 years after treatment cessation.[48] The optimal duration of denosumab treatment is unknown, and no data are available on its use in combination with other osteoporosis agents. Until more long-term data become available, denosumab should probably be reserved for patients who have not responded to bisphosphonates or cannot tolerate them.

Adverse Effects – Denosumab can lower serum calcium concentrations, especially in patients with impaired renal function; it is contraindicated for use in patients with hypocalcemia. In clinical trials, rash, eczema and dermatitis occurred more commonly with denosumab than with placebo. Rare serious infections, new malignancies and pancreatitis also occurred more often with denosumab than with placebo. Osteonecrosis of the jaw, which can occur with bisphosphonates, has been reported with denosumab. Whether long-term suppression of bone remodeling with denosumab could weaken bone rather than strengthen it is unknown.

COMBINATION THERAPY — Modest additive effects on BMD and biochemical markers of bone turnover have been demonstrated with combinations of alendronate and either estrogen or raloxifene. Whether such a combination has an additive effect in reducing the risk of fractures has not been established. There is also a concern that combination treatment with 2 different antiresorptive agents could oversuppress bone turnover and increase the risk of fractures.

One study in 126 patients already taking oral alendronate weekly found that adding a synthetic PTH (1-34) daily, or cyclically for 3 months on and 3 months off, for 15 months increased spinal BMD more than taking alendronate alone; BMD increases were similar whether PTH was given daily or intermittently.[49] In other studies, however, a bisphosphonate before PTH delayed or decreased the effects of PTH on BMD.[50,51] Raloxifene given prior to PTH may not have this effect.[52] No fracture data are available with any of these combination regimens.

Declines in BMD have been reported after PTH was discontinued; subsequent therapy with alendronate maintained the densitometric gains from PTH.[53] Subsequent treatment with raloxifene has also been shown to help prevent bone loss following PTH treatment.[54] The effect of this sequence of therapy on fracture risk has not been determined, but given the decline in BMD after cessation of PTH, many clinicians recommend following teriparatide with a bisphosphonate.

1. FRAX. WHO Fracture Risk Assessment Tool. Available at www.shef.ac.uk/FRAX. Accessed October 5, 2011.
2. RM Daly et al. Calcium- and vitamin D3-fortified milk reduces bone loss at clinically relevant skeletal sites in older men: a 2 year randomized controlled trial. J Bone Miner Res 2006; 21:397.
3. AM Grant et al. Oral vitamin D3 and calcium for secondary prevention of low-trauma fractures in elderly people (Randomised Evaluation of Calcium or Vitamin D, RECORD): a randomized placebo-controlled trial. Lancet 2005; 365:1621.
4. J Porthouse et al. Randomised controlled trial of calcium and supplementation with cholecalciferol (vitamin D3) for prevention of fractures in primary care. BMJ 2005; 330:1003.
5. RD Jackson et al. Calcium plus vitamin D supplementation and the risk of fractures. N Engl J Med 2006; 354:669.
6. HA Bischoff-Ferrari et al. Fracture prevention with vitamin D supplementation: a meta-analysis of randomized controlled trials. JAMA 2005; 293:2257.
7. BM Tang et al. Use of calcium or calcium in combination with vitamin D supplementation to prevent fractures and bone loss in people aged 50 years and older: a meta-analysis. Lancet 2007; 370:657.
8. Institute of Medicine of the National Academies. Dietary reference intakes for calcium and vitamin D. Available at http://www.iom.edu/Reports/2010/Dietary-Reference-Intakes-for-Calcium-and-Vitamin-D.aspx. Accessed October 5, 2011.
9. B Dawson-Hughes et al. IOF position statement: vitamin D recommendations for older adults. Osteoporosis Int 2010; 21:1151.
10. ML Holick et al. Evaluation, treatment, and prevention of vitamin D deficiency: an Endocrine Society clinical practice guideline. J Clin Endocrinol Metab 2011; 96:1911.

Drugs for Postmenopausal Osteoporosis

11. RB Wallace et al. Urinary tract stone occurrence in the Women's Health Initiative (WHI) randomized clinical trial of calcium and vitamin D supplements. Am J Clin Nutr 2011; 94:270.
12. J Hsia et al. Calcium/vitamin D supplementation and cardiovascular events. Circulation 2007; 115:846.
13. MJ Bolland et al. Effect of calcium supplements on risk of myocardial infarction and cardiovascular events: meta-analysis. BMJ 2010; 341:c3691.
14. MJ Bolland et al. Calcium supplements with or without vitamin D and risk of cardiovascular events: reanalysis of the Women's Health Initiative limited access dataset and meta-analysis. BMJ 2011; 342:d2040.
15. L Wang et al. Systematic review: Vitamin D and calcium supplementation in prevention of cardiovascular events. Ann Intern Med 2010; 152:315.
16. KM Sanders et al. Annual high-dose oral vitamin D and falls and fractures in older women: a randomized controlled trial. JAMA 2010; 303:1815.
17. RZ Stolzenberg-Solomon et al. Circulating 25-hydroxyvitamin D and risk of pancreatic cancer: Cohort Consortium Vitamin D Pooling Project of Rarer Cancers. Am J Epidemiol 2010; 172:81.
18. KJ Helzlsouer et al; VDDP Steering Committee. Overview of the Cohort Consortium Vitamin D Pooling Project of Rarer Cancers. Am J Epidemiol 2010; 172:4.
19. DM Black et al. Effects of continuing or stopping alendronate after 5 years of treatment: the Fracture Intervention Trial Long-term Extension (FLEX): a randomized trial. JAMA 2006; 296:2927.
20. AV Schwartz et al. Efficacy of continued alendronate for fractures in women with and without prevalent vertebral fracture: the FLEX trial. J Bone Miner Res 2010; 25:976.
21. HG Bone et al. Ten years' experience with alendronate for osteoporosis in postmenopausal women. N Engl J Med 2004; 350:1189.
22. In brief: delayed-release risedronate (Atelvia). Med Lett Drugs Ther 2011; 53:24.
23. Monthly risedronate (Actonel) for postmenopausal osteoporosis. Med Lett Drugs Ther 2008; 50:69.
24. MR McClung et al. BMD response to delayed-release risedronate 35 mg once-a-week formulation taken with or without breakfast. J Clin Densitom 2010; 13:132; Poster number 067.
25. NB Watts et al. Fracture risk remains reduced one year after discontinuation of risedronate. Osteoporos Int 2008; 19:365.
26. CH Chesnut et al. Ibandronate produces significant, similar antifracture efficacy in North American and European women: new clinical findings from BONE. Curr Med Res Opin 2005; 21:391.
27. JA Eisman et al. Efficacy and tolerability of intravenous ibandronate injections in postmenopausal osteoporosis: 2-year results from the DIVA study. J Rheumatol 2008; 35:488.
28. ST Harris et al. Ibandronate and the risk of non-vertebral and clinical fractures in women with postmenopausal osteoporosis: results of a meta-analysis of phase III studies. Curr Med Res Opin 2008; 24:237.
29. A Cranney et al. Ibandronate for the prevention of nonvertebral fractures: a pooled analysis of individual patient data. Osteoporos Int 2009; 20:291.

30. A once-yearly IV bisphosphonate for osteoporosis. Med Lett Drugs Ther 2007; 49:89.
31. DM Black et al. Once-yearly zoledronic acid for treatment of postmenopausal osteoporosis. N Engl J Med 2007; 356:1809.
32. A Grey et al. Prolonged antiresorptive activity of zoledronate: a randomized, controlled trial. J Bone Miner Res 2010; 25:2251.
33. DK Wysowski. Reports of esophageal cancer with oral bisphosphonate use. N Engl J Med 2009; 360:89.
34. B Abrahamsen et al. More on reports of esophageal cancer with oral bisphosphonate use. N Engl J Med 2009; 360:1789.
35. CR Cardwell et al. Exposure to oral bisphosphonates and risk of esophageal cancer. JAMA 2010; 304:657.
36. DK Wysowski and JT Chang. Alendronate and risedronate: reports of severe bone, joint, and muscle pain. Arch Intern Med 2005; 165:346.
37. S Fedele et al. Nonexposed variant of bisphosphonate-associated osteonecrosis of the jaw: a case series. Am J Med 2010; 123:1060.
38. M Pazianas et al. Atrial fibrillation and bisphosphonate therapy. J Bone Miner Res 2010; 25:2.
39. Reclast (zoledronic acid): Drug Safety Communication – new contraindication and updated warning on kidney impairment. Available at www.fda.gov. Accessed October 5, 2011.
40. BA Lenart et al. Atypical fractures of the femoral diaphysis in postmenopausal women taking alendronate. N Engl J Med 2008; 358:1304.
41. LY Park-Wyllie et al. Bisphosphonate use and the risk of subtrochanteric or femoral shaft fractures in older women. JAMA 2011; 305:783.
42. Raloxifene for postmenopausal osteoporosis. Med Lett Drugs Ther 1998; 40:29.
43. E Barrett-Connor et al. Effects of raloxifene on cardiovascular events and breast cancer in postmenopausal women. N Engl J Med 2006; 355:125.
44. JS Finkelstein et al. Effects of teriparatide retreatment in osteoporotic men and women. J Clin Endocrinol Metab 2009; 94:2495.
45. F Cosman et al. Retreatment with teriparatide one year after the first teriparatide course in patients on continued long-term alendronate. J Bone Miner Res 2009; 24:1110.
46. CH Chesnut III et al. A randomized trial of nasal spray salmon calcitonin in postmenopausal women with established osteoporosis: the prevent recurrence of osteoporotic fractures study. PROOF Study Group. Am J Med 2000; 109:267.
47. Denosumab (Prolia) for postmenopausal osteoporosis. Med Lett Drugs Ther 2010; 52:81.
48. HG Bone et al. Effects of denosumab treatment and discontinuation on bone mineral density and bone tumor markers in postmenopausal women with low bone mass. J Clin Endocrinol Metab 2011; 96:972.
49. F Cosman et al. Daily and cyclic parathyroid hormone in women receiving alendronate. N Engl J Med 2005; 353:566.
50. BM Obermayer-Pietsch et al. Effects of two years of daily teriparatide treatment on BMD in postmenopausal women with severe osteoporosis with and without prior antiresorptive treatment. J Bone Miner Res 2008; 23:1591.

Drugs for Postmenopausal Osteoporosis

51. S Boonen et al. Effects of previous antiresorptive therapy on the bone mineral density response to two years of teriparatide treatment in postmenopausal women with osteoporosis. J Clin Endocrinol Metab 2008; 93:852.
52. F Cosman et al. Effect of prior and ongoing raloxifene therapy on response to PTH and maintenance of BMD after PTH therapy. Osteoporos Int 2008; 19:529.
53. DM Black et al. One year of alendronate after one year of parathyroid hormone (1-84) for osteoporosis. N Engl J Med 2005; 353:555.
54. R Eastell et al. Sequential treatment of severe postmenopausal osteoporosis after teriparatide: final results of the randomized, controlled European Study of Forsteo (EUROFORS). J Bone Miner Res 2009; 24:726.

DIET, DRUGS AND SURGERY FOR
Weight Loss

Original publication date – April 2011

Adults with a body mass index (BMI=kg/m^2) of 25-<30 are considered overweight; those with a BMI of $\geq$30 are considered obese.

DIET

One pound of fat is equivalent to 3500 calories. Adults can lose 1-2 lbs (0.45-0.9 kg) of fat per week by consuming 500-1000 fewer calories per day.

COMPARATIVE TRIALS — A randomized 1-year trial in 311 non-diabetic overweight or obese pre-menopausal women (mean age 41; mean BMI 32) compared the Atkins, Zone, Ornish and LEARN diets. The only significant difference in weight loss was between the Atkins and Zone diets (4.7 vs. 1.6 kg, respectively).[1]

A randomized 2-year trial in 811 overweight adults compared 4 diets with the same degree of caloric restriction, but with different proportions of protein, fat and carbohydrate. There were no significant differences in weight loss between any of the 4 groups.[2]

A randomized 2-year trial in 307 patients (mean age 46; mean BMI 36) found that a low-carbohydrate or low-fat diet combined with intensive

Diet, Drugs and Surgery for Weight Loss

SOME COMMON DIETS

Type	Description
Weight Watchers	Moderate energy deficit Portion control
LEARN (**L**ifestyle, **E**xercise, **A**ttitude, **R**elationships, **N**utrition)	Moderate energy deficit Intensive lifestyle modification
Ornish	Vegetarian-based Fat restricted (<10% of total calories)
Zone	Low carbohydrate Carbohydrate/Protein/Fat 40/30/30
Atkins	Very low carbohydrate Minimal fat restriction

behavioral treatment resulted in weight loss of 11 kg after 1 year with either diet; after 2 years, weight loss was 6 kg with the low-carbohydrate diet and 7 kg with the low-fat diet (not a significant difference).[3]

MAINTENANCE — Patients on a diet generally lose 5% of their body weight over the first 6 months, but by 12-24 months weight often returns to baseline. The long-term ineffectiveness of weight-reduction diets may be due to compensatory changes in energy expenditure that oppose the maintenance of a lower body weight, as well as genetic and environmental factors.

In a study of 141 overweight or obese patients who achieved weight loss on a 3-month very low-calorie diet, maintenance with a high-protein diet had no benefit in decreasing weight regain after 1 year compared to a high-carbohydrate diet.[4]

In another study, 773 participants who were able to lose 11 kg on a low-calorie diet were then randomized to one of five diets. After 6 months, those on diets with a low protein content and high glycemic index regained an average of 2 kg more than those on a diet that was high in protein with a low glycemic index.[5]

Among 130 morbidly obese patients (mean BMI 44) randomized to diet plus physical activity for 1 year or diet alone for 6 months followed by diet plus physical activity for the next 6 months, the initial-activity patients lost 2% more of their baseline weight in the first 6 months (10.9 vs. 8.2 kg). At 1 year, total weight lost was 12.1 kg in the initial-activity group and 9.9 kg in those who began physical activity at 6 months.[6]

LIFESTYLE CHANGES

Lifestyle modification programs that focus on weight loss, increased physical activity and changes in energy intake can reduce the risk of type 2 diabetes.[7]

PREVENTING DIABETES — One study in 3234 non-diabetic patients (mean age 51; mean BMI 34) with fasting and post-load serum glucose elevations found that lifestyle changes over approximately 3 years were more effective in preventing diabetes than treatment with metformin (*Glucophage*, and others) (29% incidence with placebo, 22% with metformin, 14% with lifestyle changes).[7] Another 3-year study of lifestyle changes in 1079 patients with a BMI $\geq$24 and an impaired glucose tolerance test found that each kg of weight loss produced a 16% reduction in diabetes risk.[8] In one follow-up study, the reduced risk of developing diabetes as a result of weight loss intervention was found to persist for up to 20 years.[9]

IN DIABETES — A randomized 4-year trial in 5145 overweight or obese patients with type 2 diabetes found that intensive lifestyle intervention focusing on caloric restriction and increased physical activity was more successful than traditional diabetes support and education in achieving and maintaining significant weight loss and in improving hemoglobin A_{1C}, blood pressure, HDL-cholesterol and triglycerides.[10]

DRUGS

FDA-APPROVED — Only a few drugs are FDA-approved for treatment of obesity (see Table), and all have major drawbacks. Pharmacotherapy for weight loss should probably be reserved for patients with a BMI >30 or a BMI >27 plus a co-morbidity such as hypertension or diabetes.

Sympathomimetic amines – The oldest weight-loss drugs are sympathomimetic amines such as methamphetamine, phentermine and diethylpropion. All of these are classified as controlled substances. Phentermine was widely used with fenfluramine until the combination ("phen-fen") was found to be associated with heart valve abnormalities.[11] Fenfluramine and dexfenfluramine, a related drug, were found to cause valvular heart disease and primary pulmonary hypertension and were removed from the market.

Drugs in this class are approved only for short-term (up to 12 weeks) use; short-term use of phentermine or diethylpropion was associated with a mean weight loss of about 3 kg more than with placebo.[12] Data on adverse events in weight-loss trials that used sympathomimetic amines are limited, but include increases in heart rate and blood pressure, dry mouth, nervousness, insomnia and constipation.

Orlistat *(Xenical; Alli)* – Available both over the counter and by prescription, orlistat is a pancreatic and gastric lipase inhibitor that decreases absorption of fat from the gastrointestinal tract.[13] Used as an adjunct to diet, it is modestly effective in increasing weight loss. Patients taking orlistat 120 mg three times daily for 1-4 years have lost about 2.5-3.2 kg more than those taking a placebo.[14] Adverse effects including flatulence with discharge, oily spotting and fecal urgency occur predominantly after high-fat dietary indiscretions and are associated with a high incidence of drug discontinuation. Rare cases of severe liver injury have been reported

FDA-APPROVED DRUGS FOR TREATMENT OF OBESITY[1]

Drug	Some Available Formulations	Usual Daily Dosage
SYMPATHOMIMETIC AMINES[2,3]		
Benzphetamine –		
generic	25, 50 mg tabs	25-50 mg once[4]
Didrex (Pfizer)	50 mg tabs	to 50 mg tid
Diethylpropion –		
generic	25 mg tabs	25 mg tid[5]
Tenuate (Aventis)		
controlled-release –		
Tenuate Dospan (Aventis)	75 mg ER tabs	75 mg once[6]
Methamphetamine –		
generic	5 mg tabs	5 mg bid-tid[7]
Desoxyn (Ovation)		
Phendimetrazine –		
generic	35 mg tabs	35 mg bid-tid
Bontril PDM (Valeant)		to 70 mg tid[5]
extended-release –		
generic	105 mg ER caps	105 mg once[8]
Bontril (Valeant)		
Phentermine –		
generic	15, 30, 37.5 mg caps, 37.5 mg tabs	5-37.5 mg once[6]
Adipex-P (Gate)	37.5 mg tabs, caps	37.5 mg once[6]
OTHERS		
Orlistat –		
Xenical (Roche)	120 mg caps	120 mg tid[10]
Alli [9]	60 mg caps	60 mg tid[10]

1. Weight loss drugs including OTC medications are not recommended for use during pregnancy.
2. Approved only for short-term use (a few weeks).
3. Do not take within 2 weeks of starting or stopping a monoamine oxidase (MAO) inhibitor.
4. Usually taken mid-morning to mid-afternoon.
5. Taken one hour before meals.
6. Usually taken mid-morning.
7. Taken 30 minutes before meals. Not recommended for anorectic use in children <12 years old.
8. Taken 30-60 minutes before breakfast.
9. Available OTC.
10. Taken with fatty meals or up to 1 hour later; omit dose if meal is skipped; approved for up to 2 years' use. Diet should contain <30% fat.

in patients taking orlistat; a cause and effect relationship has not been established. Fat-soluble vitamin supplements should be taken 2 hours before or after taking orlistat.[15]

OFF-LABEL — Antidepressants – Serotonin is believed to play a role in regulation of satiety. Some reports have suggested that patients who take fluoxetine (*Prozac*, and others), sertraline (*Zoloft*, and others), paroxetine (*Paxil*, and others) or other **selective serotonin reuptake inhibitors (SSRIs)** for depression tend to lose weight. Clinical trials have confirmed that these drugs can increase weight loss in the first 6-12 months of a calorie-restricted diet, but long-term use of SSRIs can lead to weight gain, with some patients becoming heavier than they were at baseline. Other adverse effects include nervousness, insomnia and sexual dysfunction.

Bupropion (*Wellbutrin SR*, and others) is a non-SSRI antidepressant also used for treatment of tobacco dependence (as *Zyban*).[16] In a 24-week randomized, double-blind trial, patients (mean BMI 36) who took 300 or 400 mg of bupropion SR daily achieved weight loss of 7.2% and 10.1%, respectively, compared to a loss of 5% with placebo.[17] Bupropion is generally well tolerated; it has been reported to increase the risk of seizures, but the sustained-release formulation is less likely to have this effect. Insomnia and anxiety can occur.

In a randomized, controlled 56-week trial, combination therapy with **sustained-release bupropion and the opioid receptor antagonist naltrexone** was more effective in promoting weight loss (5-6%, depending on the naltrexone dose) than placebo (1.3% weight loss) in 1453 overweight or obese participants. Only 50% of patients completed the trial, and the patients who took the active drug had more nausea, headache, dizziness, constipation, dry mouth and vomiting than those randomized to placebo.[18] As an adjunct to behavioral modification therapy for weight loss, a combination of bupropion SR 360 mg/day and naltrexone SR 32 mg/day was associated with an additional 4% weight reduction compared to placebo in 407 patients who completed a randomized 56-week trial.

Nausea was more frequent in the combination therapy arm than with placebo.[19] A fixed-dose combination of bupropion and naltrexone (*Contrave*) was recently denied approval by the FDA because of a lack of long-term data demonstrating cardiovascular safety.

Antiepileptics – In a randomized 16-week trial, 30 patients with a mean BMI of 36 who took gradually increasing doses of **zonisamide (*Zonegran*, and others)** to a maximum of 600 mg per day as an adjunct to diet lost an average of 5.9 kg, compared to an average of 0.9 kg lost in 30 patients on placebo.[20] Zonisamide has caused dizziness, cognitive problems such as confusion, difficulty concentrating and speech abnormalities, increases in serum creatinine concentrations, and fatal Stevens-Johnson syndrome.[21]

In a 60-week trial, 854 obese patients who took **topiramate (*Topamax*, and others)** doses of 96, 192 and 256 mg daily achieved loss of 7.0%, 9.1% and 9.7%, respectively, of their baseline body weight compared to a 1.7% loss with placebo.[22] In a 16-week placebo-controlled study of 111 obese patients (BMI $\geq$27) with type 2 diabetes on a diet alone or in combination with metformin, controlled-release topiramate titrated to 175 mg per day produced significant weight loss compared to placebo (6.0 vs. 2.5 kg), but with high rates of neurological and psychiatric adverse events including paresthesias, somnolence, and difficulties in memory, concentration and attention.[23]

Antidiabetics – Metformin (*Glucophage*, and others), a biguanide marketed for oral treatment of type 2 diabetes, has produced modest weight loss in some patients, including patients with impaired glucose metabolism ("pre-diabetes") and those who take antipsychotic medications that cause weight gain.[7,24,25] Metformin can cause unpleasant gastrointestinal effects, including metallic taste, nausea, diarrhea and abdominal pain.[26]

Exenatide (*Byetta*), a glucagon-like peptide-1 (GLP-1) agonist that stimulates glucose-dependent insulin secretion, is FDA-approved as an adjunct to oral agents for treatment of type 2 diabetes.[27] Given twice

Diet, Drugs and Surgery for Weight Loss

daily by subcutaneous injection for 30 weeks, it caused dose-dependent reductions in weight (1.6-2.8 kg, compared to placebo) in patients with type 2 diabetes also taking metformin or a sulfonylurea.[28,29] In 152 non-diabetic obese patients with impaired glucose metabolism, exenatide for 24 weeks in conjunction with lifestyle modification produced a 5.1-kg weight loss compared to a 1.6-kg loss with placebo.[30] Pancreatitis and renal insufficiency have been reported with exenatide.[31]

Liraglutide (*Victoza*), a once-daily injectable GLP-1 agonist,[32] caused more weight loss (4.8-7.2 kg, dose- dependent) than placebo (2.8 kg) and orlistat (4.1 kg) in an open-label, 20-week trial in 564 obese patients (BMI 30-40) without diabetes. Nausea and emesis were the main adverse effects.[33]

Pramlintide (*Symlin*), an amylin analog given by subcutaneous injection before meals at the same time as insulin, can also produce weight loss.[34] A 16-week randomized trial in 204 obese patients (mean BMI 38), including 20% with type 2 diabetes, found that pramlintide 240 mcg three times daily was associated with a 3.7% placebo-corrected weight loss.[35] Pramlintide 120 mcg three times daily, or 240 mcg or 360 mcg 2 or 3 times daily, was more effective than placebo in preventing weight regain after an initial 4-month trial of weight loss in 411 obese patients without diabetes. Weight loss at month 12 was 6-7 kg (dose-dependent) with pramlintide, while patients on placebo regained all the weight they had lost.[36] Adverse effects included nausea, irritation at the injection site and mild hypoglycemia.

Exenatide, **liraglutide** and **pramlintide** all slow gastric emptying and may slow or decrease absorption of oral drugs.

OTHER DRUGS — **Sibutramine** (*Meridia*), a norepinephrine and serotonin reuptake inhibitor used for weight loss in adults with either type 2 diabetes or cardiovascular disease was associated with an increased risk of cardiovascular events[37] and was withdrawn from the US market. **Rimonabant**, a cannabanoid type 1 receptor antagonist associ-

282

ated with weight loss and psychiatric adverse effects, was not approved by the FDA. **Lorcaserin**, an experimental 5-HT2c serotonin receptor agonist, produced an average weight loss of 5.8 kg in 1595 obese or overweight patients, but drop-out rates were high (45%).[38] Headache, dizziness and nausea were the most common adverse effects of the drug. **Human chorionic gonadotropin** (hCG; *Novarel*, *Pregnyl* and others) is sold on the internet for sublingual use, even though it is not absorbed from the GI tract. A meta-analysis of 24 trials concluded that there was no scientific evidence that taking hCG by any route is effective for treatment of obesity.[39] Used in combination with pramlintide, **metreleptin**, an experimental leptin analog, has been reported to cause satiety and modest weight loss.[40] It has not been reviewed by the FDA.

SURGERY

Surgical treatment for obesity is generally limited to patients with a BMI >40 or a BMI >35 with an obesity-related co-morbidity, who are willing to modify their diet and increase their physical activity. However, the FDA recently approved use of the *Lap Band* for gastric banding in patients with a BMI as low as 30 with an obesity-related co-morbidity.

ROUX-EN-Y GASTRIC BYPASS — A mixed restrictive and malabsorptive procedure, Roux-en-Y gastric bypass creates a proximal 20-30 mL pouch of stomach and anastomoses it to a limb of jejunum, bypassing most of the stomach, all of the duodenum and the first 15-20 cm of the jejunum. Undigested nutrients meet digestive enzymes in the common channel where the two separated limbs join.

Efficacy – The mean loss of excess weight with this procedure has been 65-75%. Resolution or improvement rates for diabetes have been about 86%, for hypertension 79%, and for hyperlipidemia about 70%.[41] A large retrospective cohort study suggested a 40% reduction in all-cause mortality, including death from diabetes, cardiovascular disease and cancer, in patients who had undergone gastric bypass surgery compared to a severely obese control population, but the incidence of death related to accidents or suicide was higher in the surgical group.[42]

Adverse Effects – In a prospective, non-randomized study of 30-day outcomes, perioperative mortality for Roux-en-Y gastric bypass surgery was 0.2% when performed laparoscopically (n=2975), and 2.1% with an open procedure (n=437). The composite end-point of death, deep vein thrombosis (DVT) or venous thromboembolism (VTE), reintervention or hospital stay over 30 days occurred more commonly with open than with laparoscopic procedures (7.8 vs. 4.8%).[43] Iron, calcium, vitamin D and vitamin B_{12} deficiency can occur because of malabsorption. Dumping syndrome (nausea, bloating, colic, diarrhea) can occur because of rapid emptying from the gastric pouch into the jejunum. Some patients who had a gastric bypass developed clinically significant hyperinsulinemic hypoglycemia; the pathophysiology remains unclear.[44]

ADJUSTABLE GASTRIC BANDING — Use of an adjustable gastric band placed laparoscopically around the proximal portion of the stomach and injected with variable amounts of saline has now largely replaced fixed gastric banding. If patients continue to feel hungry or are not losing weight at an expected rate, they can receive an outpatient injection of saline through a subcutaneous reservoir to help increase restriction and promote satiety.

Efficacy – Data on gastric banding are confounded by studies that have combined non-adjustable with adjustable gastric bands. Loss of excess weight is about 47.5% with co-morbidity resolution or improvement rates of up to 47.9%.[41] In a meta-analysis of 129 studies focusing on two specific adjustable gastric band devices (adjustable gastric band and *Lap Band*) used in 28,980 patients, improvement or resolution rates were about 60% for type 2 diabetes and 43-63% for hypertension.[45]

Adverse Effects – Adjustable gastric banding is a restrictive procedure with no associated malabsorption; the 30-day perioperative mortality rate was 0% in 1198 patients undergoing laparoscopic banding, while the composite rate of death, DVT or VTE, reintervention or hospital stay over 30 days was 1%.[46] Slippage, band erosion, excess vomiting and port site and tubing problems are the most common adverse effects; these may require an operative revision.

SLEEVE GASTRECTOMY — Sleeve gastrectomy is a laparoscopic partial gastrectomy, in which most of the greater curvature of the stomach is removed resulting in a tubular stomach. It is now a primary procedure for patients with a higher BMI who might not achieve weight loss goals with bypass or banding.[47] Sleeve gastrectomy and gastric bypass may result in more weight loss than gastric banding, but gastric banding appears to be safer.[46]

OUTCOMES — In a large review of 2235 obese patients with type 2 diabetes who required medication for their diabetes before any type of weight reduction surgery, 75% of patients were off medication at 6 months after surgery and 85% had stopped their diabetes medication by 2 years.[48]

In a 10-year prospective, non-randomized trial in 4047 obese participants, maximal weight loss (32% with gastric bypass and 20% with gastric banding) occurred at 1-2 years in the 2010 patients who had surgery. After 10 years, weight loss stabilized at 25% with gastric bypass and at 14% with gastric banding. Mortality (adjusted for sex, age and risk factors) was 29% lower in patients who had surgery compared to those who received conventional treatment.[49] A meta-analysis of 44,022 patients from 8 clinical trials of gastric bypass or adjustable gastric banding found reductions in all-cause mortality (OR 0.70) and cardiovascular mortality (OR 0.58) in surgically treated patients compared to obese controls.[50]

CONCLUSION

Losing even a small amount of weight and increasing physical activity can prevent some of the complications of obesity, particularly type 2 diabetes. Diet and exercise are the preferred methods for losing weight, but are still associated with high long-term failure rates. Drugs may help some patients, but few effective drugs are available for weight reduction. Gastric surgery along with diet and exercise can produce marked weight loss in the obese, while significantly reducing obesity related co-morbidities; long-term data on safety are encouraging but limited.

1. CD Gardner et al. Comparison of the Atkins, Zone, Ornish, and LEARN diets for change in weight and related risk factors among overweight premenopausal women: the A to Z Weight Loss Study: a randomized trial. JAMA 2007; 297:969.

2. FM Sacks et al. Comparison of weight-loss diet with different compositions of fat, protein, and carbohydrates. N Engl J Med 2009; 360:859.

3. GD Foster et al. Weight and metabolic outcomes after 2 years on a low-carbohydrate versus low-fat diet: a randomized trial. Ann Intern Med 2010; 153:147.

4. EA Delbridge et al. One-year weight maintenance after significant weight loss in healthy overweight and obese subjects: does diet composition matter? Am J Clin Nutr 2009; 90:1203.

5. TM Larsen et al. Diets with high or low protein content and glycemic index for weight-loss maintenance. N Engl J Med 2010; 363:2102.

6. BH Goodpaster et al. Effects of diet and physical activity interventions on weight loss and cardiometabolic risk factors in severely obese adults: a randomized trial. JAMA 2010; 304:1795.

7. WC Knowler et al [Diabetes Prevention Program Research Group]. Reduction in the incidence of type 2 diabetes with lifestyle intervention or metformin. N Engl J Med 2002; 346:393.

8. RF Hamman et al. Effect of weight loss with lifestyle intervention on risk of diabetes. Diabetes Care 2006; 29:2102.

9. G Li et al. The long-term effect of lifestyle interventions to prevent diabetes in the China Da Qing Diabetes Prevention Study: a 20-year follow-up study. Lancet 2008; 371:1783.

10. The Look AHEAD Research Group. Long-term effects of a lifestyle intervention on weight and cardiovascular risk factors in individuals with type 2 diabetes mellitus: four-year results of the Look AHEAD trial. Arch Intern Med 2010; 170:1566.

11. H Jick. Heart valve disorders and appetite-suppressant drugs. JAMA 2000; 283:1738.

12. Z Li et al. Meta-analysis: pharmacologic treatment of obesity. Ann Intern Med 2005; 142:532.

13. In brief: Orlistat OTC for weight loss. Med Lett Drugs Ther 2007; 49:49.

14. D Rucker et al. Long-term pharmacotherapy for obesity and overweight: updated meta-analysis. BMJ 2007; 335:1194.

15. Orlistat for obesity. Med Lett Drugs Ther 1999; 41:55.

16. Drugs for tobacco dependence. Treat Guidel Med Lett 2008; 6:61.

17. JW Anderson et al. Bupropion SR enhances weight loss: a 48-week double-blind, placebo-controlled trial. Obes Res 2002; 10:633.

18. FL Greenway et al. Effect of naltrexone plus bupropion on weight loss in overweight and obese adults (COR-I): a multicentre, randomised, double-blind, placebo-controlled, phase 3 trial. Lancet 2010; 376: 595.
19. TA Wadden et al. Weight loss with naltrexone SR/bupropion SR combination therapy as an adjunct to behavior modification: The COR-BMOD Trial. Obesity (Silver Spring) 2011; 19:110.
20. KM Gadde et al. Zonisamide for weight loss in obese adults: a randomized controlled trial. JAMA 2003; 289:1820.
21. Zonisamide (Zonegran) for epilepsy. Med Lett Drugs Ther 2000; 42:94.
22. J Wilding et al. A randomized double-blind placebo-controlled study of the long-term efficacy and safety of topiramate in the treatment of obese subjects. Int J Obes Relat Metab Disord 2004; 28:1399.
23. J Rosenstock et al. A randomized, double-blind, placebo-controlled, multicenter study to assess the efficacy and safety of topiramate controlled release in the treatment of obese type 2 diabetic patients. Diabetes Care 2007; 30:1480.
24. RR Wu et al. Lifestyle intervention and metformin for treatment of antipsychotic-induced weight gain: a randomized trial. JAMA 2008; 299:185.
25. L Maayan et al. Effectiveness of medications used to attenuate antipsychotic-related weight gain and metabolic abnormalities: a systematic review and meta-analysis. Neuropsychopharmacology 2010; 35:1520.
26. Metformin/repaglinide (Prandimet) for type 2 diabetes. Med Lett Drugs Ther 2009; 51:41.
27. Exenatide (Byetta) for type 2 diabetes. Med Lett Drugs Ther 2005; 47:45.
28. JB Buse et al. Effects of exenatide (Exendin-4) on glycemic control over 30 weeks in sulfonylurea-treated patients with type 2 diabetes. Diabetes Care 2004; 27:2628.
29. RA DeFronzo et al. Effects of exenatide (Exendin-4) on glycemic control and weight over 30 weeks in metformin-treated patients with type 2 diabetes. Diabetes Care 2005; 28:1092.
30. J Rosenstock et al. Effects of exenatide and lifestyle modification on body weight and glucose tolerance in obese subjects with and without pre-diabetes. Diabetes Care 2010; 33:1173.
31. In brief: exenatide (Byetta) for weight loss. Med Lett Drugs Ther 2006; 48:21.
32. Liraglutide (Victoza) for type 2 diabetes. Med Lett Drugs Ther 2010; 52:25.
33. A Astrup et al. Effects of liraglutide in the treatment of obesity: a randomised, double-blind, placebo-controlled study. Lancet 2009; 374: 1606.
34. Pramlintide (Symlin) for diabetes. Med Lett Drugs Ther 2005; 47:43.
35. L Aronne et al. Progressive reduction in body weight after treatment with the amylin analog pramlintide in obese subjects: a phase 2, randomized, placebo-controlled dose-escalation study. J Clin Endocrinol Metab 2007; 92:2977.
36. SR Smith et al. Sustained weight loss following 12-month pramlintide treatment as an adjunct to lifestyle intervention in obesity. Diabetes Care 2008; 31:1816.
37. WP James et al. Effect of sibutramine on cardiovascular outcomes in overweight and obese subjects. N Engl J Med 2010; 363:905.
38. SR Smith et al. Multicenter, placebo-controlled trial of lorcaserin for weight management. N Eng J Med 2010; 363:245.

39. GK Lijesen et al. The effect of human chorionic gonadotropin (HCG) in the treatment of obesity by means of the Simeons therapy: a criteria-based meta-analysis. Br J Clin Pharmacol 1995; 40:237.
40. E Ravussin et al. Enhanced weight loss with pramlintide/metreleptin: an integrated neuro-hormonal approach to obesity pharmacotherapy. Obesity (Silver Spring) 2009; 17:1736.
41. H Buchwald et al. Bariatric surgery: a systematic review and meta-analysis. JAMA 2004; 292:1724.
42. TD Adams et al. Long-term mortality after gastric bypass surgery. N Engl J Med 2007; 357:753.
43. The Longitudinal Assessment of Bariatric Surgery (LABS) Consortium. Perioperative safety in the longitudinal assessment of bariatric surgery. N Engl J Med 2009; 361:445.
44. GJ Service et al. Hyperinsulinemic hypoglycemia with nesidioblastosis after gastric-bypass surgery. N Engl J Med 2005; 353:249.
45. SA Cunneen et al. Studies of Swedish adjustable gastric band and lap-band: systematic review and meta-analysis. Surg Obes Relat Dis 2008; 4:174.
46. NJ Birkmeyer et al. Hospital complication rates with bariatric surgery in Michigan. JAMA 2010; 304:435.
47. Clinical Issues Committee of the American Society for Metabolic and Bariatric Surgery. Updated position statement on sleeve gastrectomy as a bariatric procedure. Surg Obes Relat Dis 2010; 6:1.
48. MA Makary et al. Medication utilization and annual health care costs in patients with type 2 diabetes mellitus before and after bariatric surgery. Arch Surg 2010; 145:726.
49. L Sjöström et al. Effects of bariatric surgery on mortality in Swedish obese subjects. N Eng J Med 2007; 357:741.
50. AE Pontiroli et al. Long-term prevention of mortality in morbid obesity through bariatric surgery. a systematic review and meta-analysis of trials performed with gastric banding and gastric bypass. Ann Surg 2011; 253:484.

Index

Index

Index

Index

Index

Index

Index

Index

Index

Index

Index

Index